Third Edition

Critical Care

C E R T I F I C A T I O N
PRACTICE EXAMS

Thomas Ahrens, RN, DNS, CCRN
Clinical Specialist in Critical Care
Barnes Hospital
St. Louis, Missouri

Donna Prentice, RN, MSN, CCRN
Clinical Specialist in Critical Care
Barnes Hospital
St. Louis, Missouri

APPLETON & LANGE
Norwalk, Connecticut

0-8385-1250-X

Copyright © 1993 by Appleton & Lange
Simon & Schuster Business and Professional Group
Previous editions © 1991, © 1983 by Appleton & Lange

93 94 95 96 97 / 10 9 8 7 6 5 4 3 2 1

Prentice Hall International (UK) Limited, *London*
Prentice Hall of Australia Pty. Limited, *Sydney*
Prentice Hall Canada, Inc., *Toronto*
Prentice Hall Hispanoamericana, S.A., *Mexico*
Prentice Hall of India Private Limited, *New Delhi*
Prentice Hall of Japan, Inc., *Tokyo*
Simon & Schuster Asia Pte. Ltd., *Singapore*
Editora Prentice Hall do Brasil Ltda., *Rio de Janeiro*
Prentice Hall, *Englewood Cliffs, New Jersey*

Library of Congress Cataloging-in-Publication Data

Ahrens, Thomas.
    Critical care : certification practice exams / Thomas Ahrens,
Donna Prentice. — Ed. 3.
        p.   cm.
    ISBN 0-8385-1250-X
    1. Intensive care nursing—Examinations, questions, etc.
I. Prentice, Donna. II. Title.
    [DNLM: 1. Critical Care—examination questions. 2. Critical Care—
nurses' instruction. WY 18 A287c 1993]
    RT120.I5A39 1993
    610.73'61'076—dc20
    DNLM/DLC   92-48542
    for Library of Congress   CIP

PRINTED IN THE UNITED STATES OF AMERICA

Acknowledgments

We wish to thank Mary Ellen Frantz, RN, MSN, CCRN;
Kim Tucker, RN, BSN, CCRN; and Shawn E. Ray, RN, BSN, CCRN,
for their help in preparing and
reviewing questions for accuracy.

Contents

Part III: Answers to Practice Exams

Preface

This practice examination text is designed to complement the textbook, *Critical Care: Certification Preparation and Review, 3rd edition*. All test questions in this text are based on information in the textbook. Both texts have been revised to more accurately reflect the content on the CCRN examination.

Questions are intended to teach you as well as prepare you for the CCRN test material. Questions are organized to reflect each conceptual area tested and are structured in a manner similar to the CCRN examination questions. Approximately four times the number of questions are provided in the practice sections as you will see on the test. Any of these questions are fair game for the CCRN test. The sample tests at the end of the practice examinations provide only a sample of the types of questions you may see on the examination as no test will exactly duplicate the CCRN test. In our experience, if you can achieve approximately a 70 percent correct response rate on the final practice examination, your chances of passing the CCRN examination are fairly good.

This text adheres closely to the CCRN test blueprint. It includes the types of questions on the CCRN examination, such as recall, comprehension, and situational level questions. The practice examinations have more basic questions than the actual CCRN examination, and this is done in an attempt to help you develop a good foundation of knowledge in each content area. The final practice test, however, is more closely related to the actual CCRN test structure.

In preparing for the CCRN examination, start your preparation a few weeks before the test. Identify the areas in which you have difficulty and study them carefully. In order to pass the examination, you must do well throughout the test, as poor performance in a few areas can cause failure. The CCRN failure rate has traditionally been high with countless nurses missing a passing score by a small amount. You may avoid a near miss if your greatest preparation is in those areas in which you are less skilled. Also, prepare for the areas that receive the greatest coverage on the CCRN examination, such as cardiovascular, pulmonary, and multisystem patient-care problems. Do not, however, study only these major areas. If you have difficulty in any test area, read the text *Critical Care: Certification Preparation and Review, 3rd edition*, which is designed to accompany this practice examination book.

As you prepare for the examination, the best way to remember material is to use your knowledge in practice settings. This accomplishes two key goals: the retention of information (for the purpose of the CCRN examination) and the improvement of your patient care skills (improving your clinical skills). We believe if you try to apply material you are studying, the value of the test will be far greater than the successful achievement of the CCRN status. Your improvement in practice will be an equally valuable asset.

In this edition, we have also added another comprehensive practice exam. This allows you to take the exam once, prepare again, and then retake the second exam. In addition, we have tried to reference the answers to locations in *Critical Care: Certification Preparation & Review*. These references are intended to help you understand why a particular answer was given. Not all questions are specifically addressed in these references but most are clearly explained.

No text is perfect, and no text can provide a perfect replica of the CCRN test to prepare you for the examination. If you find flaws in the test items or have suggestions for questions, changes, or improvements, please feel free to write. We would very much appreciate any comments. Good luck in preparing for the CCRN examination!

Thomas Ahrens, RN, DNS, CCRN
Donna Prentice, RN, MSN, CCRN

Test-Taking Tips

The following are some general test-taking tips. Follow them as you prepare for the examinations in this text and on the CCRN examination. They can make the difference in several points on the examination.

1. Answer all questions. Unanswered questions are counted as incorrect.

2. Be well rested before the examination. Get a good night's sleep before the examination. Do not try to "cram" the morning of the test; you may confuse yourself if you study right before the test.

3. Have a good but light breakfast. You will be taking the test for perhaps 4 hours. Eat food that is not all carbohydrates to make it through the examination without becoming hungry or getting a headache.

4. Do not change answers unless you are absolutely sure: most first impressions are accurate.

5. Go through the test and answer all questions. Mark on a piece of scrap paper questions that are difficult. Then go back and review the difficult questions. Do not be discouraged if there are many hard questions.

6. Do not expect to answer all questions correctly. If you really do not know the answer, make a guess and go on. Do not let it bother you because you know you missed a few. You really do not have a good perception of how you did until you get the results.

7. Do not let the fact that other people finish early (or that you finish before others) disturb you. People work at different rates without necessarily a difference in results.

8. If you feel thirsty or need to go to the restroom, ask permission from the monitor. Always try to maintain your physiological status at optimal levels. An aspirin (or similar analgesic) may be in order if a headache develops during the test.

9. Do not try to establish patterns in how the items are written (for example, "Two B's have occurred, now some other choice is likely."). The AACN Certification Corporation has excellent test-writing mechanisms. Patterns in test answers, if they occur, would be coincidental.

PART 1

Practice Exams

CHAPTER 1 _____

Cardiovascular Practice Exam

1. The PCWP (pulmonary capillary wedge pressure) is an estimation of which factor regulating stroke volume?

    (A) preload
    (B) afterload
    (C) contractility
    (D) capillary permeability

2. Which two valves are normally closed during systole?

    (A) aortic and pulmonic
    (B) pulmonic and tricuspid
    (C) tricuspid and aortic
    (D) mitral and tricuspid

3. Which two valves are normally open during systole?

    (A) aortic and pulmonic
    (B) pulmonic and tricuspid
    (C) tricuspid and aortic
    (D) mitral and tricuspid

4. Which of the following is the best location at which to detect a systolic murmur due to mitral regurgitation?

    (A) second ICS (intercostal space), left of sternum
    (B) second ICS, right of sternum
    (C) fourth ICS, left of sternum
    (D) fifth ICS, midclavicular line

5. What is the approximate normal left atrial (PCWP, pulmonary capillary wedge pressure) value?

    (A) 0 to 5 mm Hg
    (B) 5 to 10 mm Hg
    (C) 8 to 12 mm Hg
    (D) 12 to 18 mm Hg

6. What is the approximate normal right atrial CVP (central venous pressure) value?

(A) 0 to 5 mm Hg
(B) 5 to 10 mm Hg
(C) 8 to 12 mm Hg
(D) 12 to 18 mm Hg

7. Which of the following is the outermost lining of the heart?

(A) endocardium
(B) myocardium
(C) transcardium
(D) pericardium

8. Which of the following statements regarding the coronary sinus is correct?

(A) It provides arterial blood flow to the lateral left ventricular wall.
(B) It provides arterial blood flow to the sinus node.
(C) It is the main venous drainage vessel of the heart.
(D) It stimulates secretion of the atrial naturietic factor.

9. Left atrial pressure approximates which pressure?

(A) pulmonary mean pressure
(B) left ventricular end diastolic pressure
(C) right atrial pressure
(D) CVP (central venous pressure)

10. Of the following four factors, three determine stroke volume. Identify the factor that does NOT affect stroke volume.

(A) preload
(B) afterload
(C) contractility
(D) mean arterial pressure

11. Which of the following are atrioventricular valves?

(A) mitral and tricuspid
(B) pulmonic and aortic
(C) mitral and aortic
(D) tricuspid and pulmonic

12. The A wave on the CVP (central venous pressure) and PCWP (pulmonary capillary wedge pressure) tracing represents which physical event?

    (A) ventricular filling
    (B) atrial contraction
    (C) atrial filling
    (D) tricuspid and mitral valve movement

13. The Y descent on the CVP (central venous pressure) and PCWP (pulmonary capillary wedge pressure) tracing occurs due to which anatomic event?

    (A) pulmonic and tricuspid valve closure
    (B) aortic and mitral valve opening
    (C) mitral and tricuspid valve closure
    (D) mitral and tricuspid valve opening

14. What is the normal right ventricular end diastolic pressure?

    (A) 0 to 5 mm Hg
    (B) 5 to 10 mm Hg
    (C) 10 to 15 mm Hg
    (D) >20 mm Hg

15. Which of the following is an estimate of right ventricular preload?

    (A) pulmonary capillary wedge pressure
    (B) central venous pressure
    (C) pulmonary artery mean pressure
    (D) coronary sinus pressure

16. Afterload is estimated by which parameter?

    (A) CVP (central venous pressure)
    (B) PCWP (pulmonary capillary wedge pressure)
    (C) stroke volume
    (D) SVR (systemic vascular resistance)

17. Which hemodynamic waves are produced by the atria?

    (A) A, C, and V waves
    (B) arterial systolic waves
    (C) augmented diastolic waves
    (D) X, Y, and Z waves

18. Left ventricular (LV) failure alone presents with all but one of the following signs. Select the INCORRECT sign.

    (A) increased CVP (central venous pressure)
    (B) increased PCWP (pulmonary capillary wedge pressure)
    (C) increased LV end diastolic pressure
    (D) increased pulmonary mean arterial pressure

19. Two circumstances may produce a systolic murmur. One exists when backward flow of blood (regurgitant flow) occurs through a valve that is normally closed during systole. The second exists when blood has difficulty getting past a valve (stenosis) that is normally easily opened. Which two situations may produce a systolic murmur?

    (A) aortic stenosis and mitral regurgitation
    (B) pulmonic regurgitation and tricuspid stenosis
    (C) aortic and tricuspid stenosis
    (D) pulmonic and mitral regurgitation

20. Which part of the ECG (electrocardiogram) correlates to a diastolic murmur?

    (A) PR interval
    (B) QRS complex
    (C) ST segment
    (D) post-T wave

21. The PCWP (pulmonary capillary wedge pressure) is used to estimate which of the following pressures?

    (A) left atrial pressure and left ventricular end diastolic pressure
    (B) right atrial pressure and right ventricular end diastolic pressure
    (C) central venous and pulmonary arterial pressures
    (D) mean pulmonary artery and right ventricular peak pressures

22. Pericardial tamponade presents with all but one of the following symptoms. Identify the symptom NOT associated with pericardial tamponade.

    (A) equalization of left and right atrial pressures [CVP (central venous pressure) and PCWP (pulmonary capillary wedge pressure)]
    (B) left ventricular failure without right ventricular involvement
    (C) hypotension
    (D) distended neck veins

23. Left ventricular preload is estimated from all of the following pressures but one. Identify the one pressure that does NOT permit one to estimate left ventricular preload.

(A) CVP (central venous pressure)
(B) PCWP (pulmonary capillary wedge pressure)
(C) left atrial pressure
(D) left ventricular end diastolic pressure

24. Right ventricular failure is manifested by which of the following signs?

(A) increased CVP (central venous pressure)
(B) increased PCWP (pulmonary capillary wedge pressure)
(C) decreased pulmonary artery pressure
(D) increased systemic arterial pressure

Questions 25 and 26 refer to the following scenario.

A 62-year-old male is admitted to your unit with the diagnosis of acute subendocardial infarction. He presently has no chest pain and vital signs are normal. As you are talking with him, he complains of sudden, severe shortness of breath. His blood pressure is 80/50, pulse 118, respiratory rate 34. Heart sounds are easily heard but he has a new systolic murmur, grade V/VI. Hemodynamic data indicate the following:

PA	38/25
PCWP	24
CVP	7
CO	3.2
CI	1.7

25. Based on the preceding information, which condition is likely to be developing?

(A) pericardial tamponade
(B) mitral valve rupture
(C) ventricular wall rupture
(D) aortic valve rupture

26. Which treatment would be indicated for this condition?

(A) immediate surgery
(B) dopamine and nipride
(C) fluid challenges
(D) thrombolytic therapy

27. Dysfunction of the papillary muscle producing mitral regurgitation would be seen in which part of the left atrial PCWP (pulmonary capillary wedge pressure) tracing?

    (A) giant A waves
    (B) absent A waves
    (C) giant C waves
    (D) giant V waves

28. Phase 0 of cellular impulse transmission refers to which phase of electrical action?

    (A) depolarization
    (B) early repolarization
    (C) end repolarization
    (D) myocardial relaxation

29. Spontaneous diastolic depolarization occurs during which phase of the cardiac action potential?

    (A) phase 0
    (B) phase 1
    (C) phase 3
    (D) phase 4

30. Which electrolyte is responsible for initial depolarization?

    (A) sodium
    (B) potassium
    (C) chloride
    (D) calcium

31. Which cation activates the second (slow channel) inward flow of ions during cardiac depolarization?

    (A) sodium
    (B) potassium
    (C) chloride
    (D) calcium

32. Which ion leaves the cell during depolarization to counter the inward flow of sodium?

    (A) phosphate
    (B) potassium
    (C) chloride
    (D) calcium

33. Which of the following cardiac chambers contains deoxygenated blood?

(A) right ventricle
(B) left ventricle
(C) pulmonary veins
(D) left atrium

34. Where is the SA (sinoatrial) node located?

(A) right atrium
(B) left atrium
(C) right ventricle
(D) superior vena cava

35. Which component of blood pressure regulation has the strongest effect on controlling the blood pressure?

(A) stroke volume
(B) cardiac output
(C) systemic vascular resistance
(D) mean arterial pressure

36. Which of the following corresponds most closely to the normal ejection fraction?

(A) 10 to 20%
(B) 25 to 35%
(C) 40 to 50%
(D) >60%

37. Starling's law refers to which of the following relationships?

(A) As fluid fills the lungs, gas exchange decreases.
(B) As coronary blood flow increases, preload falls.
(C) As afterload increases, stroke volume improves.
(D) As muscle stretches, contraction strength increases.

38. Normally, at approximately which PCWP (pulmonary capillary wedge pressure) does lung water begin to accumulate?

(A) 8 to 12 mm Hg
(B) 12 to 18 mm Hg
(C) >18 mm Hg
(D) PCWP pressure does not correlate with lung water

39. Which of the following is the most common reason for the PCWP (pulmonary capillary wedge pressure) and CVP (central venous pressure) to increase?

(A) left and right ventricular failure
(B) excess blood volume
(C) right ventricular failure
(D) pulmonary hypertension

40. Reduction of myocardial oxygen consumption is best achieved through which of the following changes?

(A) reducing afterload
(B) reducing preload
(C) increasing contractility
(D) increasing preload

41. Which neurologic structure or system has the strongest effect on regulating the heart rate?

(A) sympathetic nervous system
(B) parasympathetic nervous system
(C) adrenergic system
(D) cerebellum

42. Which of the following could produce giant A waves?

(A) aortic stenosis
(B) mitral regurgitation
(C) mitral stenosis
(D) hypovolemia

43. Posterior hemiblock is seen when which conduction defect occurs?

(A) obstruction of the left main bundle branch
(B) obstruction of the right main bundle branch
(C) blockage of the posterior portion of the right bundle
(D) blockage of the posterior portion of the left bundle

44. What is the preferred first treatment for ventricular fibrillation?

(A) CPR (cardiopulmonary resuscitation)
(B) lidocaine, 1 mg/kg
(C) synchronized cardioversion, 50 to 100 joules
(D) defibrillation, 200 to 300 joules

45. Which of the the following leads are used in the diagnosis of an inferior MI (myocardial infarction)?

(A) V_1, V_2, V_3, V_4
(B) I, aVL
(C) V_5, V_6
(D) II, III, aVF

46. Which of the following leads are used in the diagnosis of an anterior MI (myocardial infarction)?

(A) V_1, V_2, V_3, V_4
(B) I, aVL
(C) V_5, V_6
(D) II, III, aVF

47. Which of the the following leads are used in the diagnosis of a lateral MI (myocardial infarction)?

(A) V_1, V_2, V_3, V_4
(B) I, aVL, V_5, V_6
(C) V_{2R}, V_{3R}, V_{4R}
(D) II, III, aVF

48. Which of the the following leads are used in the diagnosis of a right ventricular MI (myocardial infarction)?

(A) V_1, V_2, V_3, V_4
(B) I, aVL, V_5, V_6
(C) aVR, aVL, aVF
(D) V_1, V_2, V_{4R}, V_{6R}

49. An atrial premature beat with aberrant conduction usually has which of the following characteristics?

(A) left bundle branch block
(B) left anterior hemiblock
(C) right bundle branch block
(D) posterior hemiblock

50. Interpret the following ECG rhythm strip. Sinus rhythm with:

    (A) left ventricular PVC (premature ventricular contraction)
    (B) APC (atrial premature contraction) with aberrant conduction
    (C) right ventricular PVC
    (D) interpolated PVC

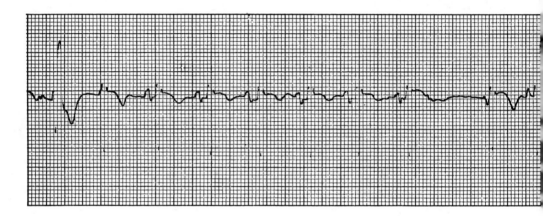

51. Interpret the following ECG rhythm strip.

    (A) sinus tachycardia
    (B) atrial tachycardia
    (C) atrial flutter
    (D) atrial fibrillation

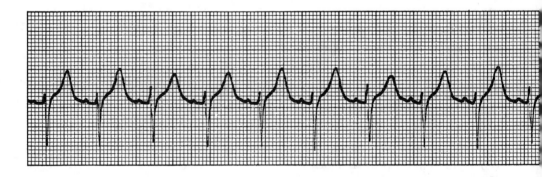

52. Interpret the following ECG rhythm strip.

    (A) sinus tachycardia
    (B) atrial tachycardia
    (C) atrial flutter
    (D) atrial fibrillation

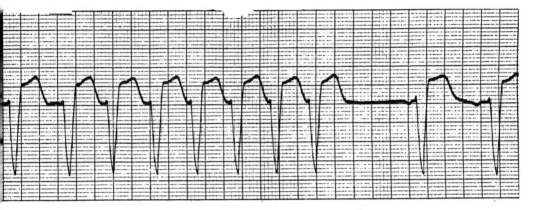

53. Interpret the following ECG rhythm strip.

    (A) sinus tachycardia
    (B) atrial tachycardia
    (C) atrial flutter
    (D) atrial fibrillation

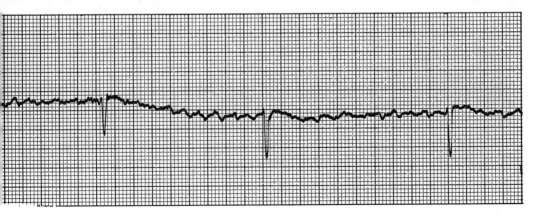

54. Interpret the following ECG rhythm strip.

   (A) sinus tachycardia
   (B) atrial tachycardia
   (C) atrial flutter
   (D) atrial fibrillation

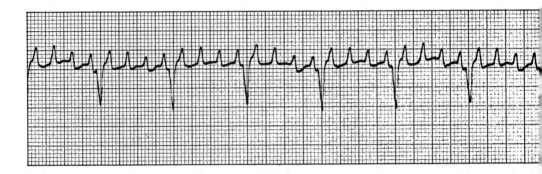

55. Interpret the following ECG rhythm strip.

   (A) first-degree block
   (B) second-degree block, type I
   (C) second-degree block, type II
   (D) third-degree block

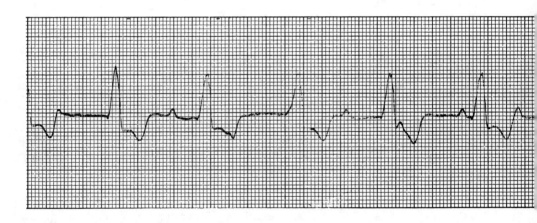

56. Interpret the following ECG rhythm strip.

    (A) first-degree block
    (B) second-degree block, type I
    (C) second-degree block, type II
    (D) third-degree block

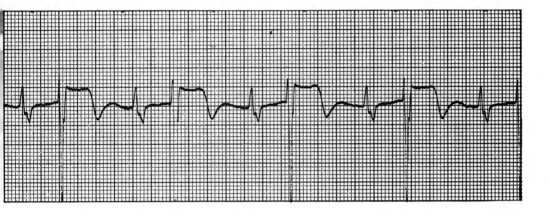

57. Interpret the following ECG rhythm strip.

    (A) first-degree block
    (B) second-degree block, type I
    (C) second-degree block, type II
    (D) third-degree block

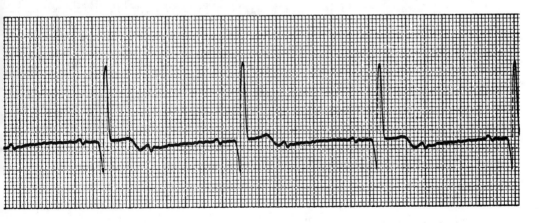

58. Interpret the following ECG rhythm strip.

   (A) first-degree block
   (B) second-degree block, type I
   (C) second-degree block, type II
   (D) third-degree block

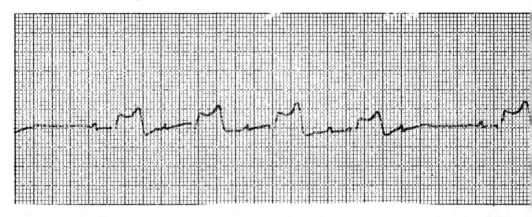

59. Interpret the following ECG rhythm strip.

   (A) multiform PVC (premature ventricular contraction)
   (B) ventricular tachycardia
   (C) ventricular fibrillation
   (D) torsade de point

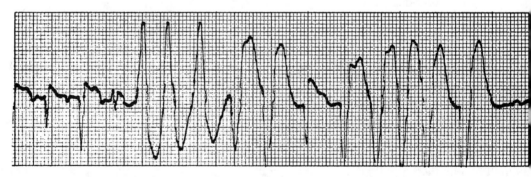

60. Interpret the following ECG rhythm strip. Atrial fibrillation with:

   (A) multiform PVC (premature ventricular contraction)
   (B) ventricular tachycardia
   (C) ventricular fibrillation
   (D) torsade de point

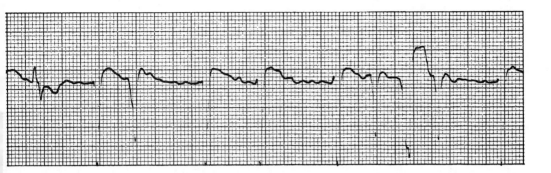

61. Interpret the following ECG rhythm strip.

(A) multiform PVC (premature ventricular contraction)
(B) ventricular tachycardia
(C) ventricular fibrillation
(D) torsade de point

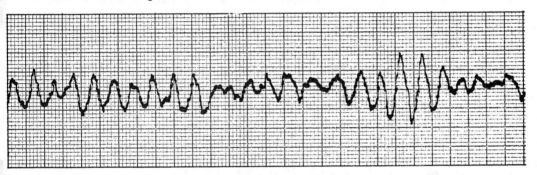

62. APCs (atrial premature contractions) with abberant conduction can be differentiated from PVCs (premature ventricular contractions) by noting ECG changes. All of the following but one are associated with PVCs rather than APCs. Identify the one associated with APCs.

(A) taller left peak (Rr') in V_1
(B) right bundle branch block
(C) marked left axis deviation
(D) rS pattern in V_6

63. Which of the following corresponds most closely to the definition of precordial concordancy?

(A) rsR' in V_1 to V_4
(B) all QRS complexes have the same axis in V_1 to V_6
(C) all T waves are inverted in V_1 to V_6
(D) left axis deviation in I and aVF

64. Inferior MIs (myocardial infarctions) produce conduction defects different from those seen in anterior MIs. Which type of dysrhythmia is more likely to occur in inferior than anterior MIs?

    (A) second-degree type I
    (B) second-degree type II
    (C) multiform PVCs (premature ventricular contractions)
    (D) APCs (atrial premature contractions) with aberrancy

65. Anterior hemiblock is manifested by which of the following 12-lead ECG patterns?

    (A) left axis deviation greater than $-30°$
    (B) right axis deviation greater than $+90°$
    (C) Q wave in V_1 to V_3
    (D) large R wave in I and aVL

66. Posterior hemiblock is manifested by which of the following 12-lead ECG patterns?

    (A) left axis deviation greater than $-30°$
    (B) right axis deviation greater than $+90°$
    (C) Q wave in V_1 to V_3
    (D) large R wave in I and aVL

67. Left ventricular hypertrophy is manifested by which of the following ECG changes?

    (A) left anterior hemiblock patterns
    (B) left bundle branch block patterns
    (C) S wave in V_1 and R wave in V_5 totaling more than 35 mm
    (D) R wave in III and S wave in aVL totaling greater than 30 mm

68. Right ventricular hypertrophy is manifested by which of the following ECG changes?

    (A) right anterior hemiblock patterns
    (B) right bundle branch block patterns
    (C) S wave in V_1 and R wave in V_5 totaling more than 35 mm
    (D) R:S ratio greater than 1:1 in V_1

69. Which of the following is NOT an example of atrioventricular (AV) dissociation?

    (A) ventricular tachycardia
    (B) third-degree heart block
    (C) first-degree heart block
    (D) atrial tachycardia with 2:1 block

70. What is the initial treatment of sinus tachycardia?

(A) verapamil
(B) initially try carotid massage, then give digoxin
(C) esmolol or Inderal
(D) There is no treatment; find the source of the tachycardia.

71. Which of the physical treatments listed below is NOT a form of parasympathetic stimulation for atrial tachycardia?

(A) carotid massage
(B) pressure on the eyeball
(C) Valsalva manuever
(D) hepatojugular reflux

Questions 72 and 73 refer to the following scenario.

A 65-year-old male is admitted to your unit with chest pain. The chest pain developed two hours ago at home. The pain went away for a while while he rested but then returned. Currently, he has substernal chest pain radiating to the left arm and chin. The pain is the same regardless of position. No change in the pain occurs during inspiration. Vital signs are as follows: blood pressure 132/86, pulse 96, respiratory rate 25. His 12-lead ECG shows depressed ST segments in the inferior leads. Small Q waves, less than one-third the height of the R wave, are present in the inferior leads.

72. Based on the preceding information, which condition is likely to be developing?

(A) angina
(B) acute myocardial infarction
(C) pericarditis
(D) pericardial tamponade

73. What would be the most likely treatment for the condition?

(A) nitrates and beta blockers
(B) thrombolytic therapy
(C) pericardiocentesis
(D) aspirin and analgesics

Questions 74 and 75 refer to the following scenario.

A 72-year-old male is admitted to your unit with the diagnosis of anterior MI (myocardial infarction). During your shift, you notice that he has developed a 2:1 heart block and a constant PR interval, with a ventricular response rate of 42. His blood pressure is 84/50.

74. Based on the preceding information and considering the type of MI (myocardial infarction), which type of heart block is likely?

(A) first-degree
(B) second-degree type I
(C) second-degree type II
(D) third-degree

75. Which treatment is likely to be most effective in stabilizing this rhythm?

(A) pacemaker
(B) calcium chloride
(C) dopamine
(D) epinephrine

76. For what does the first letter in VVI stand?

(A) ventricular paced
(B) ventricular sensed
(C) ventricular inhibited
(D) ventricular programmed

77. For what does the second letter in VVI stand?

(A) ventricular paced
(B) ventricular sensed
(C) ventricular inhibited
(D) ventricular programmed

78. In the following rhythm strip, identify the pacemaker operational state.

(A) capturing properly at 1:1
(B) failing to sense
(C) failing to capture
(D) producing pacemaker-generated ventricular ectopic beats

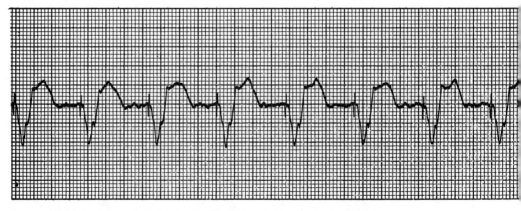

79. Which of the following is an advantage of a transcutaneous pacemaker?

(A) It is easy to apply.
(B) It requires lower electrical stimulation to capture the heart rate.
(C) It requires peripheral intravenous access.
(D) Electrical stimulation is not perceived by the patient.

Questions 80 and 81 refer to the following scenario.

A 45-year-old male is admitted to the unit with the diagnosis of inferior MI (myocardial infarction). Currently, he has no chest pain or shortness of breath. Two hours after admission, he develops a bradycardia of 50 bpm with a blood pressure of 86/54. He also develops uniform PVCs (premature ventricular contractions) at the rate of ten per minute.

80. Based on the diagnosis of inferior MI (myocardial infarction), how long will the bradycardia last?

(A) It usually will be permanent and symptomatic.
(B) It usually will be transient and possibly symptomatic.
(C) Bradycardias are so uncommon with inferior MIs that some degree of CHF (congestive heart failure) must be present and the bradycardia will exist until the CHF is resolved.
(D) It usually will be permanent but asymptomatic.

81. Treatment for this dysrhythmia would most likely include which medication?

(A) lidocaine
(B) dopamine
(C) atropine
(D) epinephrine

82. What is the inherent rate of the AV (atrioventricular) node area?

(A) 20 to 40
(B) 40 to 60
(C) 60 to 80
(D) The AV node area has no inherent rate.

83. Anterior MIs (myocardial infarctions) produce conduction defects different from those seen in inferior MIs. Which type of dysrhythmia is more likely to occur in anterior than inferior MIs?

(A) APCs (atrial premature contractions) with aberrancy
(B) second-degree type I
(C) second-degree type II
(D) multiform PVCs (premature ventricular contractions)

84. Passage of the electrical impulse through the AV (atrioventricular) node is represented by which ECG complex?

(A) PR interval
(B) QRS complex
(C) ST segment
(D) T wave

85. Atrial tachycardia is intially treated with which pharmacologic agent?

(A) atropine
(B) verapamil
(C) digitalis
(D) inderal

Questions 86 and 87 refer to the following scenario.

A 66-year-old female is admitted to your unit with the diagnosis of anterolateral MI (myocardial infarction). She has no complaints of chest pain or discomfort. While you are interviewing her, she goes into the rhythm displayed below. You ask her how she feels and she replies "I feel fine. You look worried though. Is something wrong?" Her blood pressure is 118/78.

86. What is your interpretation of the dysrhythmia?

(A) accelerated idioventricular rhythm
(B) aberrantly conducted APCs (atrial premature contractions)
(C) artifact
(D) ventricular tachycardia

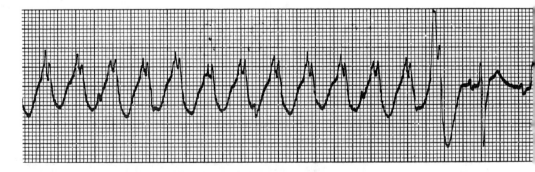

87. What would be the treatment for this rhythm?

(A) observation; no treatment necessary
(B) lidocaine
(C) synchronized defibrillation at 50 joules
(D) unsynchronized defibrillation at 200 joules

88. A junctional rhythm has all of the following characteristics but one. Which of the following characteristics is NOT indicative of a junctional rhythm?

(A) normal QRS complex
(B) wide QRS complex
(C) heart rate between 40 and 60 bpm
(D) absent P waves

89. Which lead is most likely to detect aberrantly conducted APCs (atrial premature contractions)?

(A) lead II
(B) lead III
(C) lead aVF
(D) MCL_1 lead

90. Of the following findings, all but one indicate an increased seriousness of PVCs (premature ventricular contractions). Select the factor that does NOT increase the seriousness of PVCs.

(A) uniform appearance
(B) multiform complexes
(C) PVC on T wave (R on T phenomenon)
(D) frequency greater than ten per minute

91. APCs (atrial premature contractions) with aberrant conduction can be differentiated from PVCs (premature ventricular contractions) by noting ECG changes. All of the following findings but one are associated with APCs rather than PVCs. Identify the one associated with PVCs.

(A) second R wave larger than the first in V_1
(B) right bundle branch block
(C) right axis deviation
(D) rS pattern in V_6

92. Which of the following isoenzymes is most diagnostic in identifying MI (myocardial infarction)?

(A) CPK (creatine phosphokinase)—MB band
(B) CPK—MM band
(C) CPK—BB band
(D) LDH (lactic acid dehydrogenase)—1

Questions 93 and 94 refer to the following scenario.

A 51-year-old male is admitted to your unit with the symptoms of crushing chest pain, unrelieved by nitrates or rest. He has 3-mm elevated ST segments in V_1 through V_4, with ST depression in II, III, and aVF. His blood pressure is 94/64, pulse 110, and respiratory rate 32.

93. Based on the preceding information, which type of MI (myocardial infarction) would most likely be represented by the ECG changes?

    (A) anterior
    (B) inferior
    (C) lateral
    (D) posterior

94. Is ECG confirmation of an MI (myocardial infarction) present in this patient?

    (A) no, due to the absence of Q waves
    (B) no, due to ST depression in the inferior leads
    (C) yes, due to ST segment elevation in V_1 through V_4
    (D) yes, due to absence of lateral ECG changes

95. Which type of MI (myocardial infarction) has the highest mortality rate?

    (A) anterior
    (B) inferior
    (C) lateral
    (D) posterior

96. Unstable angina is characterized by all of the following features but one. Which feature does NOT characterize unstable angina?

    (A) increasing frequency of chest pain
    (B) chest pain at rest
    (C) increasing severity of symptoms
    (D) elevation of ST segments

97. The LDH (lactate dehydrogenase) "flip," after which LDH-1 exceeds LDH-2, is potentially useful in which situation?

    (A) differentiating angina from MI (myocardial infarction)
    (B) identifying MIs in patients who present after CPK (creatine phosphokinase) levels have returned to normal
    (C) verifying the presence of Prinzmetal's angina
    (D) differentiates anterior from inferior MIs

Questions 98 through 100 refer to the following scenario.

A 65-year-old female is admitted to the unit with chest pain and MI (myocardial infarction) is ruled out. Physically, she has no shortness of breath or orthopnea, some noticeable jugular venous distension, and clear breath sounds. Her ECG shows large R waves in V_1 and V_2. Hemodynamic studies reveal the following:

blood pressure	102/72
pulse	105
PA	30/16
PCWP	13
CVP	16
CO	4.6
CI	2.4

98. Which condition is likely to be present based on the preceding information?

    (A) right ventricular hypertrophy
    (B) right ventricular infarction
    (C) left ventricular infarction
    (D) pericardial tamponade

99. What other leads may be useful in establishing a diagnosis in this patient?

    (A) MCL_1
    (B) MCL_5
    (C) aVR
    (D) V_{4R} and V_{6R}

100. Hemodynamic support would most likely include which of the following strategies:

    (A) fluids to keep the CVP (central venous pressure) elevated
    (B) diuretics to reduce the CVP
    (C) dopamine to increase the blood pressure
    (D) nitroglycerine to reduce the preload

101. Which type of medication is common in the treatment of unstable angina?

    (A) diuretics
    (B) vasodilators
    (C) beta blockers
    (D) sympathetic stimulants

Questions 102 and 103 refer to the following scenario.

A 59-year-old male is admitted to your unit with the diagnosis "rule out myocardial infarction." He stated one hour ago that he was at work when he felt severe chest pain, became cool and clammy, and felt nauseated. He came immediately to the hospital. The ECG indicates ST segment elevation in leads II, III, and aVF. ST segment depression exists in V_1 through V_6. He has not responded to nitrates in the emergency room or the intensive care unit. His vital signs are as follows:

blood pressure	98/68
pulse	107
respiratory rate	32

102. Which type of MI (myocardial infarction) is represented on the ECG changes?

    (A) anterior
    (B) inferior
    (C) lateral
    (D) posterior

103. Based on the preceding description, which initial treatment is indicated?

    (A) dobutamine
    (B) thrombolytic therapy
    (C) CABG (coronary artery bypass graft)
    (D) angioplasty

104. Thrombolytic therapy is commonly associated with complications. Which of the following is NOT a complication of thrombolytic therapy?

    (A) bradycardias
    (B) bleeding from venipuncture sites
    (C) ventricular ectopy
    (D) extension of the MI (myocardial infarction) due to embolic phenomena

105. Which of the following is an indication for angioplasty?

    (A) proximal stenosis of a coronary artery
    (B) distal stenosis of a coronary artery
    (C) multiple obstructions in coronary arteries
    (D) no prior episodes of angina

106. A patient who has failed to derive benefit from a medication regimen for unstable angina may benefit in reduction of pain from which treatment?

(A) valvuloplasty
(B) thrombolytic therapy
(C) beta blockade
(D) CABG (coronary artery bypass graft)

107. Indications for thrombolytic therapy (with optimal prognosis) include which of the following?

(A) onset of pain less than eight hours
(B) onset of pain less than four hours
(C) no prior MI (myocardial infarction)
(D) ST segment depression in two consecutive leads

108. Dopamine is used with caution in patients with MI (myocardial infarction) for which reason?

(A) its potential for increasing myocardial oxygen consumption
(B) because it has no inotropic component
(C) because it may cause reflex bradydysrhythmias
(D) due to the increase in the fibrillation threshold

109. Which of the following medications is an example of an agent that is expected to reduce directly myocardial oxygen consumption?

(A) inderal
(B) dobutamine
(C) dopamine
(D) lasix

110. Assuming vascular volume is adequate, which medication would have the strongest effect on raising the blood pressure in a hypotensive patient?

(A) norepinephrine (Levophed)
(B) dobutamine (Dobutrex)
(C) epinephrine (Adrenalin)
(D) esmolol (Brevibloc)

111. What is the stroke volume in a patient who has a cardiac output of 5.2 LPM and a heart rate of 80 bpm?

(A) 11 cc
(B) 52 cc
(C) 65 cc
(D) 101 cc

112. Pulsus paradoxus is utilized to identify which one of the following conditions?

(A) cardiac tamponade
(B) myocardial infarction
(C) respiratory failure
(D) ruptured papillary muscle

113. Orthostatic hypotension results from which of the following conditions?

(A) left ventricular failure
(B) pulmonary hypertension
(C) hypovolemia
(D) portal hypertension

114. Orthostatic hypotension is manifested by which of the following clinical symptoms following a change from lying down to sitting up?

(A) a systolic blood pressure fall of more than 25 mm Hg and a decrease in diastolic blood pressure of more than 10 mm Hg
(B) systolic blood pressure is unchanged while a decrease in diastolic blood pressure of more than 10 mm Hg occurs
(C) a decrease in systolic blood pressure while diastolic blood pressure slightly increases
(D) an increase in systolic blood pressure while diastolic blood pressure falls

115. Measurement of orthostatic hypotension occurs during measurement of blood pressure with position changes. Select the position change by means of which orthostatic hypotension should be measured.

(A) move from upright to supine
(B) move from sitting to standing
(C) move from supine to upright
(D) turn from left side to right

116. Which medication has the strongest effect (assuming normovolemia) in elevating the blood pressure?

(A) dobutamine (Dobutrex)
(B) isoproterenol (Isuprel)
(C) esmolol (Brevibloc)
(D) dopamine (Intropin)

117. Lasix is considered to affect primarily which component of stroke volume?

(A) preload
(B) afterload
(C) contractility
(D) aortic distensibility

118. Which medication promotes the largest increase in myocardial oxygen consumption (MVO_2)?

(A) nitroglycerine
(B) nitroprusside
(C) dobutamine
(D) dopamine

119. Vasodilator drugs have which of the following effects on hemodynamics?

(A) decreased SVR (systemic vascular resistance), increased PCWP (pulmonary capillary wedge pressure), decreased cardiac output
(B) increased SVR, decreased PCWP, decreased cardiac output
(C) increased CVP (central venous pressure), increased SVR, increased cardiac output
(D) decreased CVP, decreased PCWP, increased cardiac output

120. Physical signs associated with CHF (congestive heart failure) include all but one of the following. Identify the one sign that is NOT associated with CHF.

(A) dependent crackles
(B) S_3 heart sound
(C) dependent edema
(D) Kussmaul respiration

Questions 121 and 122 refer to the following scenario.

A 72-year-old male is admitted with the diagnosis of CHF (congestive heart failure). He complains of shortness of breath but does not complain of chest pain. He has bibasilar crackles and distended neck veins. His vital signs are blood pressure 112/82, pulse 110, respiratory rate 29. Pulmonary artery catheter readings reveal the following:

PA	38/23
PCWF	22
CVP	15
CO	3.6
CI	2.1

121. Based on the preceding data, which condition does this patient exhibit?

(A) left ventricular failure alone
(B) right ventricular failure alone
(C) biventricular failure
(D) chronic obstructive pulmonary disease

122. All of the following medications would be used to treat the condition but one. Identify the medication that would NOT be used for this patient.

(A) low-dose dobutamine
(B) nitroglycerine
(C) Lasix
(D) high-dose dopamine

Questions 123 and 124 refer to the following scenario.

A 68-year-old female is admitted to your unit complaining of fatigue, shortness of breath, and "swollen feet." She has the following vital signs: blood pressure 188/106, pulse 108, respiratory rate 30. Pulmonary artery catheter readings reveal the following information:

PA	42/25
PCWP	21
CVP	17
CO	3.3
CI	1.9

123. If a vasodilator were to be used in this patient, which would be the optimal agent to employ?

(A) nitroglycerine (Nitrostat)
(B) phenylephrine (Neosynephrine)
(C) Diazoxide (Hyperstat)
(D) nitroprusside (Nipride)

124. What would be the reason she has shortness of breath and fatigue?

(A) biventricular failure
(B) underlying chronic lung disease
(C) right ventricular failure
(D) pulmonary hypertension

Questions 125 and 126 refer to the following scenario.

A 75-year-old female is admitted to your unit from the emergency room with severe shortness of breath and orthopnea. She is very anxious and restless. She has a history of CHF (congestive heart failure) and was fine until this morning, when the respiratory difficulties started and became progressively worse. Her ECG shows nonspecific ST changes. Breath sounds reveal crackles throughout her lungs. Her blood pressure is 82/56, pulse 118, respiratory rate 38.

125. Based on these symptoms, which condition is probably developing?

    (A) right ventricular failure
    (B) pulmonary edema
    (C) myocardial infarction
    (D) pulmonary emboli

126. Which of the following would probably NOT be used in the treatment of this patient?

    (A) dopamine
    (B) nitroprusside
    (C) dobutamine
    (D) Lasix

127. If the physician ordered nitroprusside and dobutamine in a patient with CHF (congestive heart failure), what is the goal of this type of medication regimen?

    (A) reduced preload and improved contractility
    (B) increased preload and reduced afterload
    (C) reduced afterload and reduced contractility
    (D) reduced afterload and improved contractility

128. The use of Lasix and morphine in pulmonary edema is designed to improve myocardial function by which action?

    (A) reduce preload and myocardial oxygen consumption
    (B) reduce afterload and myocardial oxygen consumption
    (C) increase preload and improve contractility
    (D) improve contractility while increasing afterload

129. Which of the following medications is NOT a positive inotrope?

    (A) dopamine
    (B) dobutamine
    (C) amrinone
    (D) nitroprusside

130. Which of the following medications is a beta blocker?

    (A) esmolol
    (B) nifedipine
    (C) mexiletine
    (D) captopril

131. Vasodilation may help reduce myocardial oxygen consumption in the failing left ventricle. Which of the following medications produce(s) vasodilation that could be useful in the treatment of congestive heart failure?

    I. nitroprusside (Nipride)
   II. phenylephrine (Neosynephrine)
  III. nifedipine (Procardia)

        (A) I
        (B) II and III
        (C) II
        (D) I and III

132. Which of the following is NOT a calcium channel blocker?

    (A) nifedipine
    (B) diltiazem
    (C) verapamil
    (D) diazoxide

133. Pericarditis presents on the 12-lead ECG with which of the following changes?

    (A) Q waves in precordial leads
    (B) left axis deviation
    (C) generalized elevation of ST segments
    (D) depression of ST segments

134. Which of the following is NOT a symptom of pericarditis?

    (A) fever
    (B) increased pain on left lateral position
    (C) pericardial friction rub
    (D) chest pain unchanged with respiration

135. Early stages of hypovolemic or cardiogenic shock may exhibit normal blood pressure due to which of the following compensating mechanisms?

    (A) increased SVR (systemic vascular resistance)
    (B) increased preload
    (C) decreased afterload
    (D) increased stroke volume

136. Where should inflation of the balloon in an IABP (intraaortic balloon pump assist) occur?

(A) near the T wave on the ECG
(B) at end diastole
(C) at end systole
(D) near the dicrotic notch

137. Which of the following is one danger of abdominal aortic aneurysm repair?

(A) obstruction of renal blood flow
(B) interference with coronary diastolic filling
(C) creation of pulmonary emboli
(D) pericardial tamponade

138. Deflation of the balloon in an IABP (intraaortic balloon pump assist) should occur at what point?

(A) near the T wave on the ECG
(B) before the QRS complex
(C) at end systole
(D) near the dicrotic notch

139. Hypovolemic shock differs from cardiogenic shock by exhibiting which one of the following hemodynamic changes?

(A) high preload
(B) low preload
(C) high SVR (systemic vascular resistance)
(D) low stroke volume

140. Which of the following agents would most reliably raise the blood pressure in cardiogenic shock?

(A) dopamine
(B) dobutamine
(C) fluid bolus
(D) nitroprusside

141. Which of the following are two benefits of an IABP (intraaortic balloon pump assist)?

(A) decreased preload and increased afterload
(B) increased contractility and afterload
(C) decreased afterload and increased coronary filling
(D) increased coronary filling and increased preload

142. Which physical maneuver is most likely to result in improved blood pressure?

(A) placing the patient in the Trendelenburg (head-down) position
(B) sitting the patient in a semiupright position
(C) placing the patient in a prone position
(D) placing the patient in a supine position and elevating the legs

143. Which of the following is NOT a cause of hypovolemic shock?

(A) pulmonary capillary leak syndrome
(B) cardiogenic shock
(C) postoperative bleeding
(D) fracture of a long bone

144. Cardiogenic shock is characterized by which of the following parameters?

I. cardiac index less than 2.2 LPM/m²
II. PCWP (pulmonary capillary wedge pressure) greater than 22 mm Hg
III. CVP (central venous pressure) between 5 and 10 mm Hg

(A) I only
(B) I and II
(C) II and III
(D) III only

Questions 145 and 146 refer to the following scenario.

At 1600, a 67-year-old female is admitted to your unit from the emergency room with hypotension. Her husband states that she had complained of shortness of breath earlier in the day and since noon he has not been able to awaken her. She currently is unresponsive except to painful stimuli. Her blood pressure is 78/50, pulse 118. A pulmonary artery catheter is inserted and gives the following information:

PA	44/26
PCWP	25
CVP	15
CO	3.7
CI	1.6

145. Based on the preceding information, which condition is developing?

(A) cardiogenic shock
(B) hypovolemic shock
(C) right ventricular failure with pulmonary hypertension
(D) sepsis with a low SVR (systemic vascular resistance)

146. Which treatment should be initiated for this patient?

(A) fluid bolus
(B) dobutamine and dopamine
(C) lasix and nitroprusside
(D) epinephrine and lasix

Questions 147 and 148 refer to the following scenario.

A 58-year-old male is admitted to your unit with hypotension and the diagnosis "rule out myocardial infarction." He has a blood pressure of 82/52, pulse 122. During physical assessment, he exhibits marked orthopnea, extreme anxiety, and crackles throughout his lungs but more prominent posteriorly. He is to have a pulmonary artery catheter inserted in the next hour.

147. Based on these symptoms, what would you expect the hemodynamic data from the pulmonary artery catheter to reveal?

(A) PCWP less than 10, CI less than 2 L/m²
(B) PCWP greater than 22, CI less than 2 L/m²
(C) CVP greater than 15, CI greater than 4 L/m²
(D) SVR greater than 2000 dynes/sec·cm, CI greater than 4 L/m²

148. What treatment would be most effective initially for this patient?

(A) high-dose dopamine and nitroprusside
(B) lasix and morphine
(C) dobutamine and epinephrine
(D) digitalis and lasix

149. Vasoconstriction can increase the blood pressure while also increasing myocardial oxygen consumption. Which of the following drugs could be expected to produce vasoconstriction and thereby raise the blood pressure and increase MVO_2?

  I. dopamine
 II. dobutamine
III. norepinephrine

    (A) I and Il
    (B) I and III
    (C) II and III
    (D) I, II, and III

Questions 150 and 151 refer to the following scenario.

A 57-year-old male is admitted to your unit postoperatively for repair of a fractured femur and a splenectomy after a motor vehicle accident. Four hours postoperatively, his level of consciousness begins to decrease. Vital signs are as follows: blood pressure 88/58, pulse 113, respiratory rate 28. His skin is cool and clammy. He has no complaints of shortness of breath; breath sounds are clear. His pulmonary artery catheter provides the following data:

PA	21/7
PCWP	4
CVP	2
CO	3.6
CI	1.7

150. Based on the preceding information, which condition appears to be developing?

   (A) left ventricular failure
   (B) right ventricular failure
   (C) cardiogenic shock
   (D) hypovolemic shock

151. In a patient with acute blood loss, which of the following would most reliably increase the vascular volume?

   (A) NS (normal saline)
   (B) LR (lactated Ringer's)
   (C) hetastarch (Hespan)
   (D) D_5W

152. Sympathetic stimulants, such as dopamine, are not indicated in hypovolemia until the blood volume has been corrected. Which of the following is the best explanation for this approach?

   (A) Massive sympathetic stimulation is already present and cannot reach effectiveness without adequate fluid volume.
   (B) Sympathetic stimulation only works when vasodilation is the primary problem.
   (C) Sympathetic stimulation cannot occur until vascular baroreceptors have been inactivated.
   (D) Dopamine is indicated in hypovolemia before fluid replacement.

Questions 153 to 155 refer to the following scenario.

A 71-year-old female is in your unit following colon resection. Due to an episode of hypotension in the operating room, a pulmonary artery catheter was inserted. On postoperative day 1, her morning hematocrit was 35, hemoglobin 11.5. Her afternoon hematocrit is 27, hemoglobin 9. She has no complaints of pain that differ from those reported in the morning. The following are the pulmonary artery catheter readings from the morning and afternoon. She has received one liter of normal saline over the past 12 hours. The house officer is not concerned over the change, attributing the change to dilutional factors.

	MORNING	AFTERNOON
blood pressure	98/58	94/56
pulse	102	115
PA	24/12	20/8
PCWP	10	5
CVP	4	3
CO	3.9	3.7
CI	2.5	2.4

153. Based on the preceding information, which condition is developing?

   (A) The data support dilutional reasons for the drop in hematocrit and hemoglobin.
   (B) hypovolemia
   (C) left ventricular failure
   (D) pericardial tamponade

154. Which parameters best separate dilutional from actual decreases in the hematocrit and hemoglobin?

   (A) heart rate, cardiac output, and SVR (systemic vascular resistance)
   (B) stroke volume, heart rate and PCWP (pulmonary capillary wedge pressure)
   (C) PCWP and cardiac output
   (D) blood pressure and CVP (central venous pressure)

155. Why would the cardiac output not change substantially if the patient was developing hypovolemia?

   (A) The stroke volume increased to offset the loss of blood volume.
   (B) The PCWP (pulmonary capillary wedge pressure) decrease reduced myocardial oxygen consumption and improved contractility.
   (C) The heart rate increased to offset the loss of blood volume.
   (D) The mean arterial pressure increased to offset the loss of blood volume.

156. Which of the following is not an indication for a CABG (coronary artery bypass graft)?

(A) unstable angina
(B) 90% narrowing of LAD (left anterior descending coronary artery)
(C) distal stenosis of LAD
(D) multiple vessel stenosis

157. Which of the following is a common sign in cardiac tamponade?

(A) decreased PCWP (pulmonary capillary wedge pressure)
(B) increased diastolic blood pressure
(C) pulsus paradoxus
(D) ejection fraction greater than 75%

158. Which blood vessel is most commonly used as the graft vessel in a CABG (coronary artery bypass graft)?

(A) femoral vein
(B) axillary artery
(C) a coronary artery that is unobstructed
(D) internal mammary artery

159. Nursing care of the patient following cardiopulmonary bypass surgery includes observation of all of the following measures but one. Which of the following is NOT a postoperative measure for the nurse to assess?

(A) body temperature
(B) pulmonary gas exchange
(C) PT (prothrombin time)
(D) PCWP (pulmonary capillary wedge pressure) and CVP (central venous pressure)

160. Which of the following is the best method to treat cardiomyopathy?

(A) heart transplantation
(B) CABG (coronary artery bypass graft)
(C) IABP (intraaortic balloon pump assist)
(D) coronary angioplasty

161. Approximately what percent of heart transplant recipients are alive after five years?

(A) <25%
(B) 25 to 50%
(C) 50 to 75%
(D) If they survive the first year, 100% survival at five years

162. What is the most common type of aortic aneurysm?

(A) ascending thoracic
(B) descending thoracic
(C) abdominal
(D) aortic arch

163. Dissecting aneurysms present with several symptoms. Which of the following is NOT a symptom of a dissecting aortic aneurysm?

(A) gastrointestinal bleeding
(B) severe abdominal pain
(C) pain radiating to the back
(D) palpable abdominal mass

164. Dissection of an artery occurs because of which type of injury to the blood vessel?

(A) intimal tear
(B) weakness of the entire vessel wall
(C) severance of the arterial wall
(D) bleeding into an already formed aneurysm

165. Which of the following is the most common complication causing death following aortic surgery?

(A) stress ulcers
(B) ATN (acute tubular necrosis)
(C) bleeding
(D) MI (myocardial infarction)

166. All of the following but one are symptoms of obstructed arterial flow. Select the one that represents venous, NOT arterial, obstruction.

(A) pallor of the skin
(B) cyanosis of the skin
(C) intermittent claudication
(D) decreased pulses

167. Which of the following is a common sign of acute arterial obstruction?

(A) pain distal to the obstruction
(B) edema distal to the obstruction
(C) cyanosis distal to the obstruction
(D) warm skin proximal to the obstruction

168. Deep venous thrombosis can potentially release emboli. Which of the following could result from the emboli of a deep venous thrombosis?

(A) loss of dorsalis pedal pulse
(B) loss of pulses in the femoral artery
(C) superior vena caval syndrome
(D) pulmonary emboli

169. Which of the following is NOT a parameter commonly measured in a patient after a CABG (coronary artery bypass graft)?

(A) temperature
(B) PCWP (pulmonary capillary wedge pressure)
(C) cardiac output
(D) ejection fraction

Questions 170 and 171 refer to the following scenario.

A 57-year-old male is admitted to your unit following a CABG (coronary artery bypass graft). At 0400 he is alert and oriented and is extubated without difficulty. At 0500, he is lethargic despite not receiving analgesics. He has a mediastinal chest tube that has drained 500 cc in the last hour. Pulmonary artery catheter and blood gas information are listed below:

	0400	0500
blood pressure	100/70	100/66
pulse	100	110
PCWP	15	10
CVP	10	7
CO	4.3	4.0
CI	2.5	2.4
PaO_2	82	77
SaO_2	0.96	0.95
FiO_2	0.40	0.40
$PaCO_2$	37	39
pH	7.37	7.35
HCO_3-	24	23

170. Based on the preceding information, the patient is probably developing which of the following?

(A) tension pneumothorax
(B) mediastinal bleeding
(C) adult respiratory distress syndrome
(D) CHF (congestive heart failure)

171. Which treatment would be optimal for the patient at this time?

(A) initiation of dobutamine
(B) addition of epinephrine
(C) autotransfusion
(D) added pleural and mediastinal chest tubes

Questions 172 through 174 refer to the following scenario.

A 62-year-old male is admitted to your unit postoperatively following abdominal aortic aneurysm repair. Four hours after returning from the operating room, he begins to complain of chest pain and shortness of breath. Breath sounds are equal with inspiratory crackles noted posteriorly. Heart sounds indicate a clear S_1, S_2, and S_3.

172. On the basis of this information, the patient is most likely developing which of the following?

(A) MI (myocardial infarction)
(B) pulmonary emboli
(C) tension pneumothorax
(D) dissecting thoracic aneurysm

Before answering questions 173 and 174, please read the following additional information.
    Based on the development of chest pain, the patient has a pulmonary artery catheter inserted and blood gases are obtained. Analysis of this formation discloses the following:

blood pressure	96/64
pulse	112
PA	34/20
PCWP	19
CVP	11
CO	3.8
CI	2.2
PaO_2	68
SaO_2	0.92
FiO_2	0.40
$PaCO_2$	35
pH	7.40
HCO_3-	25

173. Based on the preceding information, which condition is most likely to be developing?

(A) MI (myocardial infarction)
(B) pulmonary emboli
(C) tension pneumothorax
(D) dissecting thoracic aneurysm

174. Treatment to support these hemodynamics would most likely include which of the following?

(A) fluid bolus
(B) dobutamine
(C) dopamine
(D) nitroprusside

Questions 175 through 177 refer to the following scenario.

A 68-year-old female is admitted to your unit after a CABG (coronary artery bypass graft). Eight hours following surgery, she is extubated and experiencing only mild chest discomfort. Over the next hour, she begins to complain of vaguely increasing discomfort. Her pleural tube is bubbling in the water seal chamber. No drainage is present from the mediastinal tube. Her blood pressure fluctuates with respiration, decreasing by 20 mm Hg during inspiration. Her lung sounds are clear; heart sounds are normal but distant.

175. Based on the preceding information, which condition is most likely to be developing?

(A) tension pneumothorax
(B) pneumomediastinum
(C) left ventricular failure
(D) pericardial tamponade

Before answering question 176, please read the following additional information.
A pulmonary artery catheter reveals the following information:

blood pressure	92/58
pulse	115
PA	36/22
PCWP	18
CVP	18
CO	3.2
CI	1.9

176. With the added information, does your interpretation of the situation change? Which condition is developing in this patient?

(A) tension pneumothorax
(B) dissecting aortic aneurysm
(C) pulmonary emboli
(D) cardiac tamponade

177. Which treatment would be indicated in this patient?

(A) pleural chest tube insertion
(B) insertion of a new mediastinal tube
(C) dopamine
(D) reintubation and placing the patient on postive pressure ventilation

178. Interpret the following 12-lead ECG

(A) anterior hemiblock
(B) posterior hemiblock
(C) right bundle branch block
(D) left bundle branch block

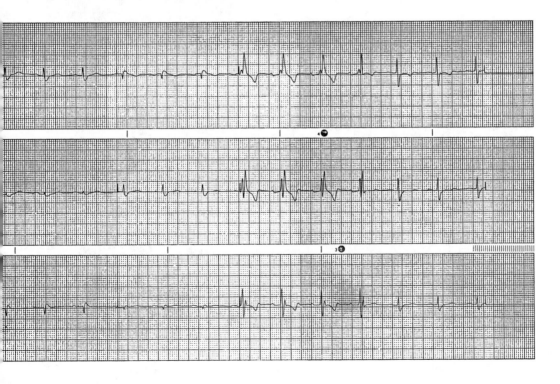

179. Interpret the following 12-lead ECG.

    (A) anterior MI (myocardial infarction)
    (B) inferior MI
    (C) posterior MI
    (D) lateral MI

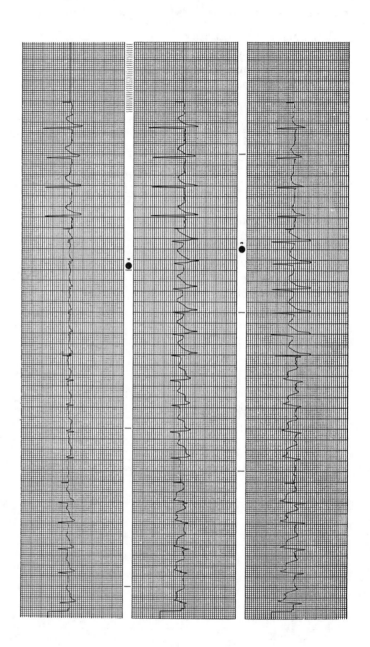

180. Interpret the following 12-lead ECG.

   (A) anterior MI (myocardial infarction)
   (B) inferior-lateral MI
   (C) posterior MI
   (D) lateral MI

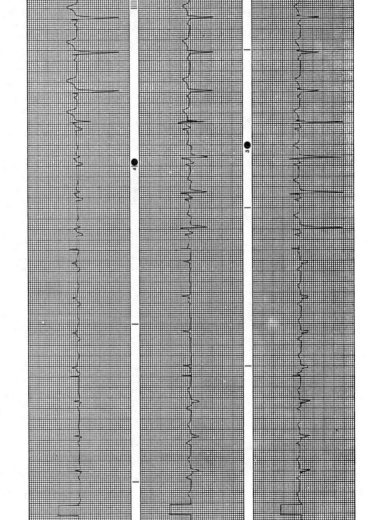

181. In the following ECG, identify the major electrocardiographic abnormality.

(A) inferior ischemia
(B) left ventricular hypertrophy
(C) right ventricular hypertrophy
(D) anterior ischemia

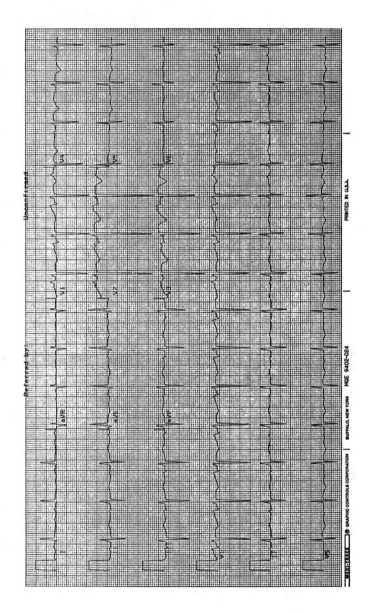

182. Interpret the following 12-lead ECG.

(A) New anterior MI (myocardial infarction)
(B) New inferior MI
(C) posterior MI
(D) anterior-inferior MI

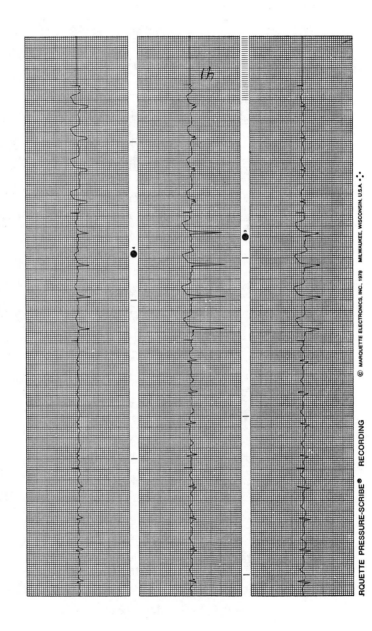

ROUETTE PRESSURE-SCRIBE® RECORDING   © MARQUETTE ELECTRONICS, INC., 1978   MILWAUKEE, WISCONSIN, U.S.A.

183. In the following ECG, identify the major electrocardiographic abnormality.

   (A) inferior ischemia
   (B) left ventricular hypertrophy
   (C) right ventricular hypertrophy
   (D) anterior ischemia

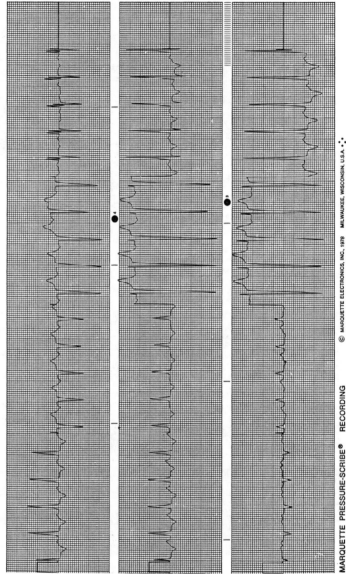

MARQUETTE PRESSURE-SCRIBE® RECORDING   © MARQUETTE ELECTRONICS, INC., 1978   MILWAUKEE, WISCONSIN, U.S.A.

184. Interpret the following 12-lead ECG.

(A) anterior hemiblock
(B) posterior hemiblock
(C) right bundle branch block
(D) left bundle branch block

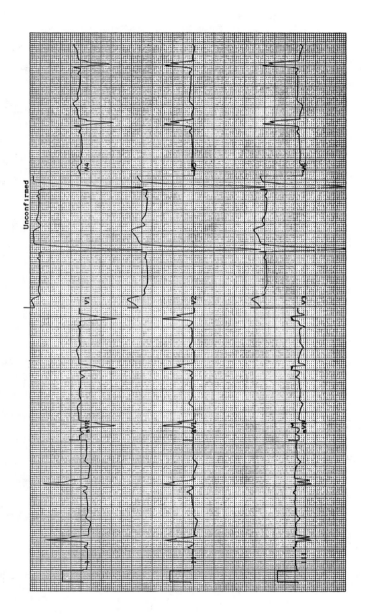

185. Interpret the following 12-lead ECG.

(A) anterior hemiblock
(B) posterior hemiblock
(C) right bundle branch block
(D) left bundle branch block

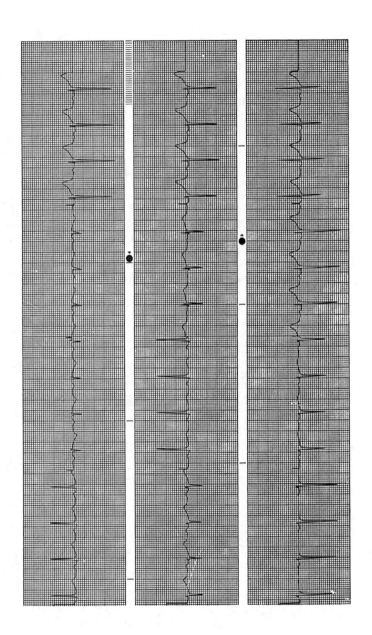

186. Which abnormality is present in the following ECG?

(A) left ventricular ectopy
(B) pericarditis
(C) left axis deviation
(D) right axis deviation

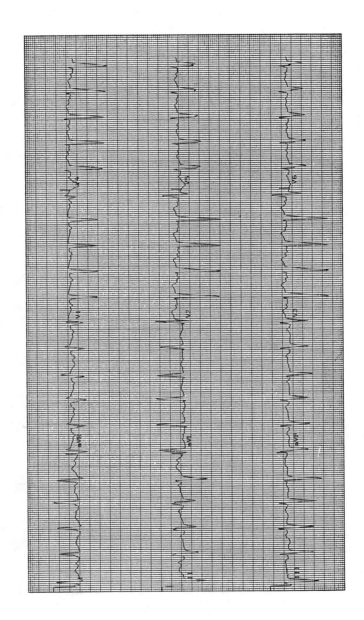

187. In the following ECG, identify the major electrocardiographic abnormality.

(A) inferior ischemia
(B) left ventricular hypertrophy
(C) right ventricular hypertrophy
(D) anteriolateral ischemia with RBBB

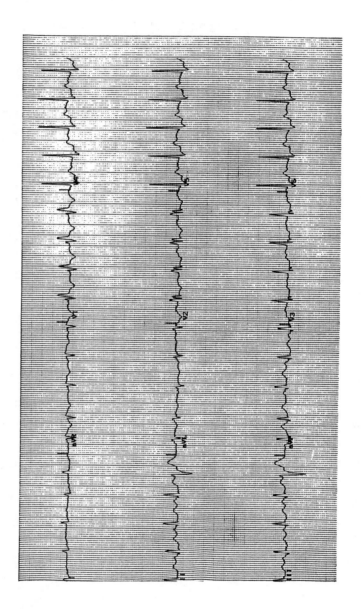

188. Interpret the following 12-lead ECG.

   (**A**) anterior hemiblock
   (**B**) atrial tachycardia with aberrancy
   (**C**) ventricular tachycardia
   (**D**) left bundle branch block

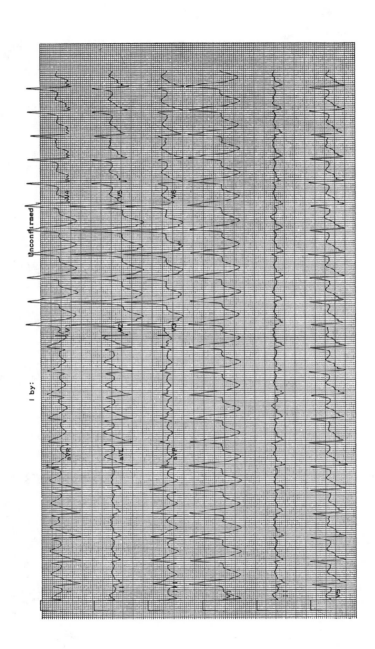

189. In the following ECG, identify the major electrocardiographic abnormality.

   (A) left bundle branch
   (B) left bundle branch block
   (C) right ventricular hypertrophy
   (D) anterior ischemia

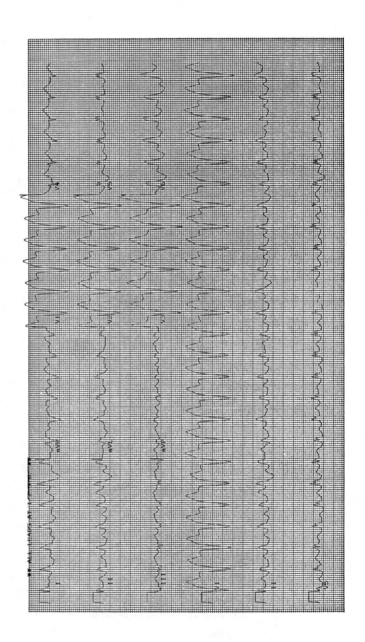

Pulmonary Practice Exam

1. The inferior border of lungs is located at which anterior (front) ICS (intercostal space)?

   (A) second ICS
   (B) fourth ICS
   (C) sixth ICS
   (D) eighth ICS

2. The superior border of the lungs is located at which anterior (front) ICS (intercostal space)?

   (A) above the clavicles
   (B) second ICS
   (C) fourth ICS
   (D) sixth ICS

3. Which statement best describes the physical relationship between both lungs and the mediastinum?

   (A) All three compartments are connected via direct air communication.
   (B) All three compartments are physically separate from each other.
   (C) The lungs are connected via communicating pleural spaces but the mediastinum is independent.
   (D) The mediastinum and right lung are connected via pleural membranes but the left lung is independent.

4. If an open pneumothorax of the right lung occurred (meaning that air could exit the lung), what would be the effect on the left lung?

   (A) The left lung would collapse.
   (B) The left lung would expand into the right lung space.
   (C) No anatomic change in the left lung would occur.
   (D) The left lung would develop atelectasis.

5. The upper airway serves three of the key functions listed below. Select the one function that is NOT served by the upper airway.

(A) humidification of air
(B) removal of particles
(C) warming of inspired air
(D) participation in gas exchange

6. Which part of the trachea is relatively avascular, allowing for emergency placement of artificial airways in this area?

(A) thyroid cartilage
(B) cricothyroid cartilage
(C) laryngopharynx
(C) glottis

7. The left and right mainstem bronchi divide from the trachea at which of the following locations?

(A) carina
(B) sternoclavicular junction
(C) lingula
(D) larynx

8. Right mainstem bronchus intubations are more likely to be performed than left bronchus intubations for which of the following reasons?

(A) The right mainstem bronchus has more ciliary clearance of mucus, facilitating passage of the endotracheal tube.
(B) The left mainstem bronchus is located several inches lower than the right.
(C) The left mainstem bronchus, although wider than the right, sits posterior to the right mainstem bronchus.
(D) The right mainstem bronchus is wider and has less angulation than the left.

9. Which part of the airways does NOT participate in gas exchange?

(A) alveoli
(B) terminal bronchioles
(C) alveolar ducts
(D) segmental bronchioles

10. What is the name of the lipoprotein secreted by alveolar type II cells that promotes alveolar expansion by increasing the surface tension of the alveoli?

   (A) surfactant
   (B) phagocytes
   (C) alveolar epithelium
   (D) pulmonary parenchyma

11. Which of the following ranges corresponds most closely to the range of normal pleural pressures?

   (A) +3 to +10
   (B)   0 to +4
   (C) −5 to +5
   (D) −3 to −8

12. The primary neurochemical control of breathing is exerted by which part of the nervous system?

   (A) pons
   (B) medulla
   (C) cerebellum
   (D) cerebral cortex

13. From which structure does the hypoxemic drive to breathe originate?

   (A) aortic and carotid arteries
   (B) pons
   (C) medulla
   (D) basal ganglia

14. Cheyne-Stokes breathing is characterized by which of the following respiratory patterns?

   (A) rapid, shallow breathing
   (B) short periods of apnea followed by respirations of increasing depth that then slow again to apnea
   (C) regular, deep breathing patterns that alternate with shallow breathing patterns over a period of several minutes
   (D) slow, deep breaths

15. Which of the following best describes the purpose of the Hering-Breuer (stretch) reflex?

(A) prevention of overdistension of the lung
(B) prevention of atelectasis
(C) stimulation of the hypoxemic drives to breathe
(D) regulation of respiratory rate and depth

16. Intubation of the esophagus may occur during attempts to intubate the trachea. Why is the esophagus easier to intubate than the trachea?

(A) The trachea is behind the esophagus.
(B) The posterior pharynx transition to the esophagus creates a natural path.
(C) The trachea is less distensible and remains in a collapsed position until inspiration occurs.
(D) The esophagus can be intubated due to the presence of the cricoid cartilage, which directs objects into the esophagus rather than the trachea.

17. In order to avoid ischemia of the trachea during endotracheal intubation, endotracheal cuff pressures should remain below venous drainage pressures. Normal venous pressures in the trachea fall within which of the following ranges?

(A) 0 to 5 mm Hg
(B) 5 to 10 mm Hg
(C) 10 to 15 mm Hg
(D) 15 to 20 mm Hg

18. Normal arterial PO_2 levels (at sea level) fall within which of the following ranges?

(A) 20 to 35 mm Hg
(B) 35 to 45 mm Hg
(C) 60 to 80 mm Hg
(D) 80 to 100 mm HG

19. Normal venous PO_2 levels (at sea level) fall within which of the following ranges?

(A) 20 to 35 mm Hg
(B) 35 to 45 mm Hg
(C) 60 to 80 mm Hg
(D) 80 to 100 mm Hg

20. Normal arterial hemoglobin saturation (SaO_2) fall within which of the following ranges?

(A) 0.40 to 0.60
(B) 0.60 to 0.80
(C) 0.80 to 0.90
(D) >0.95

21. Normal mixed venous hemoglobin saturation (SvO_2) fall within which of the following ranges?

(A) 0.40 to 0.60
(B) 0.60 to 0.75
(C) 0.80 to 0.90
(D) >0.95

22. When comparing finger oximetry values (SpO_2) to SaO_2 levels, which of the following statements is most accurate?

(A) SpO_2 values underestimate SaO_2 values.
(B) SpO_2 values overestimate SaO_2 values.
(C) SpO_2 values should equal SaO_2 values.
(D) SpO_2 values do not correlate with SaO_2 values.

23. When measuring how easily the lungs distend, which of the following is the best method to estimate distensibility?

(A) static compliance
(B) dynamic compliance
(C) diffusion gradients
(D) PEEP (positive end expiratory pressure) compliance measurements

24. When measuring the elastic recoil of the lungs, which of the following is the best method to employ?

(A) static compliance
(B) dynamic compliance
(C) mouth occlusion pressures
(D) capnography tests

25. Which of the following does NOT worsen dynamic compliance?

(A) obesity
(B) airway secretions
(C) third-trimester pregnancy
(D) loss of airway rigidity

26. Which of the following best describes vital capacity?

(A) maximal inspiration followed by maximal expiration
(B) normal inspiratory volumes
(C) the amount of air vital to the person in one minute
(D) the amount of air in the lungs at rest

27. The amount of air that does NOT participate in gas exchange is referred to by which of the following terms?

(A) minute ventilation
(B) alveolar ventilation
(C) dead space ventilation
(D) bronchial ventilation

28. Alveolar ventilation is described by which of the following formulas?

(A) dead space ventilation + tidal volume
(B) minute volume − dead space ventilation
(C) tidal volume + minute ventilation
(D) respiratory rate × tidal volume

29. Which level of dead space is considered normal?

(A) 25 to 35%
(B) 40 to 50%
(C) 55 to 65%
(D) 70 to 80%

Questions 30 and 31 refer to the following scenario.

A 28-year-old female is admitted with acute shortness of breath. Her respiratory rate is 39 bpm, V_T 500 cc, pulse 126, blood pressure 140/88. She has a history of asthma and is compliant with her medication regime. Her blood gases reveal the following information:

PaO_2	71
$PaCO_2$	27
pH	7.50
HCO_3-	24

30. Based on the preceding information, what would you estimate her dead space to be?

(A) normal
(B) probably low
(C) probably elevated
(D) The dead space cannot be estimated based on blood gases and minute ventilation.

31. What is her minute ventilation?

    (A) elevated
    (B) low
    (C) normal
    (D) The minute ventilation cannot be estimated.

32. Which of the following is the most common cause of hypoxemia?

    (A) diffusion barriers
    (B) hypoventilation
    (C) changes in barometric pressure
    (D) intrapulmonary shunts

33. Which of the following is an estimate of intrapulmonary shunting?

    (A) arterial/alveolar ratio
    (B) diffusion capacity
    (C) mixed venous oxygen tensions
    (D) FEV_1 (forced expiratory volume in one second)

34. Which of the following is the best description of FIO_2 (fraction of inspired oxygen)?

    (A) the molecular weight of oxygen
    (B) the percent of oxygen during inspiration
    (C) the amount of oxygen (in cc) during inspiration
    (D) the fraction of oxygen versus carbon dioxide during inspiration

35. Which of the following would be a normal oxygen tension (PaO_2) on exposure to 100% oxygen?

    (A) 60 to 100 mm Hg
    (B) 100 to 250 mm Hg
    (C) 250 to 400 mm Hg
    (D) 400 to 600 mm Hg

Questions 36 and 37 refer to the following scenario.

A 48-year-old male is admitted with the diagnosis of noncardiogenic pulmonary edema. Analysis of his blood gases reveals the following:

PaO_2	86
$PaCO_2$	36
pH	7.37
FIO_2	50%

36. Estimate the intrapulmonary shunt from the preceding data.

(A) normal
(B) low
(C) elevated
(D) The pulmonary shunt cannot be estimated if the patient is on oxygen.

37. Assume that the patient is on a regular diet. Based on the preceding data would it be safe to remove his oxygen in order to allow him to eat?

(A) no
(B) yes
(C) only if his nutritional status was depleted
(D) yes, providing he rests during the meal

38. Normal intrapulmonary shunts fall within which of the following ranges?

(A) 0 to 5%
(B) 6 to 15%
(C) 16 to 21%
(D) >21%

39. Which of the following is the most important determinant of oxygen transport?

(A) PaO_2
(B) SaO_2
(C) hemoglobin level
(D) cardiac output

40. Which of the following is an indicator of the balance between oxygen transport and consumption?

(A) PaO_2
(B) SaO_2
(C) SvO_2
(D) oxygen delivery

Questions 41 and 42 refer to the following scenario.

A 62-year-old female is admitted to the unit with respiratory failure following hip replacement surgery. She complains of shortness of breath and orthopnea. She has the following laboratory data available:

PaO$_2$	61
SaO$_2$	0.90
SvO$_2$	0.65
PaCO$_2$	39
pH	7.35
FIO$_2$	60%

41. Based on the preceding information, which condition is likely to be developing?

    (A) severe intrapulmonary shunt
    (B) severe imbalance between oxygen transport and cellular oxygen demand
    (C) increased oxygen extraction rates
    (D) hypercarbic respiratory failure

42. Does the FIO$_2$ need to be increased, based on her oxygenation status?

    (A) No, the SvO$_2$ indicates adequate oxygenation.
    (B) Yes, the PaO$_2$ is low and warrants further oxygen therapy.
    (C) Yes, the SvO$_2$ is low and warrants further oxygen therapy.
    (D) No, since her intrapulmonary shunt is near normal.

43. If the SvO$_2$ level decreases, all of the following parameters but one should be investigated by the nurse. Which parameter does NOT warrant investigation?

    (A) oxygen content (CaO$_2$)
    (B) SMA-6 (electrolytes)
    (C) cardiac output
    (D) oxygen consumption

44. Which of the following corresponds most closely to the normal oxygen transport level?

    (A) 250 to 550 cc/min
    (B) 600 to 1000 cc/min
    (C) 1200 to 1600 cc/min
    (D) 1600 to 2000 cc/min

45. Which of the following exerts the primary chemical control over breathing?

    (A) oxygen tension
    (B) carbonic acid level
    (C) carbon dioxide level
    (D) bicarbonate level

46. Which of the following corresponds most closely to the normal minute ventilation (V_E)?

   (A) 1 to 4 LPM
   (B) 5 to 10 LPM
   (C) 11 to 15 LPM
   (D) >15 LPM

47. The oxyhemoglobin dissociation curve is best described as illustrating which of the following?

   (A) the ability of oxygen to dissociate into different ions
   (B) the amount of oxygen carried in the blood per minute
   (C) the amount of oxygen carried in the dissolved state
   (D) the ability of hemoglobin to bind with oxygen

48. An acid is best described as which of the following?

   (A) a substance that gives up a hydrogen ion
   (B) a substance that accepts a hydrogen ion
   (C) an entity preventing oxygen from taking the electron cleaved from hydrogen
   (D) a substance that depletes free floating hydrogen from the blood

49. The pulmonary response to a change in hydrogen ion concentration occurs in which time frame?

   (A) within 24 hours
   (B) within 48 hours
   (C) within one week
   (D) within five minutes

50. The renal response to a change in hydrogen ion concentration occurs in which time frame?

   (A) within 24 hours
   (B) within 48 hours
   (C) within one week
   (D) within five minutes

51. Which of the following is the basis for the primary renal buffering mechanism for a change in hydrogen ion level?

   (A) bicarbonate
   (B) phosphate
   (C) protein
   (D) sulfate

Questions 52 through 57 require you to interpret a set of blood gas values.

52. What would be the correct interpretation of the following blood gas values?

pH   7.35
PaCO$_2$ 72
HCO$_3$−   41

(A) respiratory acidosis alone
(B) respiratory acidosis with compensating metabolic alkalosis
(C) metabolic alkalosis alone
(D) metabolic acidosis with compensating respiratory alkalosis

53. What would be the correct interpretation of the following blood gas values?

pH   7.22
PaCO$_2$ 64
HCO$_3$−   24

(A) respiratory acidosis alone
(B) respiratory acidosis with compensating metabolic alkalosis
(C) metabolic alkalosis alone
(D) metabolic acidosis with compensating respiratory alkalosis

54. What would be the correct interpretation of the following blood gas values?

pH   7.53
PaCO$_2$ 36
HCO$_3$−   35

(A) respiratory acidosis alone
(B) respiratory acidosis with compensating metabolic alkalosis
(C) metabolic alkalosis alone
(D) metabolic acidosis with compensating respiratory alkalosis

55. What would be the correct interpretation of the following blood gas values?

pH   7.55
PaCO$_2$ 21
HCO$_3$−   26

(A) respiratory alkalosis alone
(B) respiratory alkalosis with compensating metabolic acidosis
(C) metabolic alkalosis alone
(D) metabolic acidosis with compensating respiratory alkalosis

56. What would be the correct interpretation of the following blood gas values?

pH	7.36
$Paco_2$	24
HCO_3-	14

(A) respiratory alkalosis alone
(B) respiratory alkalosis with compensating metabolic alkalosis
(C) metabolic alkalosis alone
(D) metabolic acidosis with compensating respiratory alkalosis

57. What would be the correct interpretation of the following blood gas values?

pH	7.15
$Paco_2$	37
HCO_3-	11

(A) respiratory acidosis alone
(B) respiratory acidosis with compensating metabolic alkalosis
(C) metabolic acidosis alone
(D) metadolic acidosis with compensating respiratory alkalosis

Questions 58 and 59 refer to the following scenario.

A 58-year-old male admitted with the diagnosis of COPD (chronic obstructive pulmonary disease) presents with shortness of breath, circumoral cyanosis, and orthopnea. He is alert and oriented, stating that these symptoms started a few days earlier. He presents with the following blood gas values:

pH	7.36
$Paco_2$	66
Pao_2	50
HCO_3-	37
FIo_2	room air

58. Based on the preceding information, which condition is likely to be developing?

(A) acute oxygenation failure
(B) acute ventilation failure
(C) metabolic acidosis
(D) pure respiratory acidosis

59. Which treatment would be indicated for this patient?

(A) intubation and mechanical ventilation
(B) PEEP (positive end expiratory pressure) therapy
(C) inverse ratio ventilation
(D) high-flow, low-FIO_2 oxygen therapy

60. A patient with the diagnosis of asthma is admitted to your unit. He has received initial bronchodilator therapy in the emergency room. His blood gas values at that time were as follows:

pH	7.39
$PaCO_2$	25
PaO_2	62
HCO_3-	25
FIO_2	0.30

Which of the following sets of blood gas values would indicate a worsening of the asthmatic episode due to diminished alveolar air flow?

(A) pH 7.30, $PaCO_2$ 48, PaO_2 70, FIO_2 0.40
(B) pH 7.35, $PaCO_2$ 29, PaO_2 69, FIO_2 0.40
(C) pH 7.48, $PaCO_2$ 18, PaO_2 60, FIO_2 0.40
(D) pH 7.39, $PaCO_2$ 24, PaO_2 58, FIO_2 0.40

61. Which of the following parameters is used as an estimate of alveolar ventilation (V_A)?

(A) PaO_2
(B) $PaCO_2$
(C) pH
(D) alveolar-arterial oxygen gradient

62. At which pH is an acidosis generally treated?

(A) <7.25
(B) 7.25 to 7.35
(C) 7.35 to 7.45
(D) any pH greater than 7.45

63. Which of the following is NOT a cause of acute respiratory failure?

(A) CNS (central nervous system) injury
(B) right ventricular failure
(C) excessive use of narcotics
(D) left ventricular failure

64. Excessive extravascular lung water is normally removed from the pulmonary interstitial compartment by which of the following?

(A) alveolar type III cells
(B) increasing plasma osmotic pressure
(C) decreasing plasma hydrostatic pressure
(D) pulmonary lymphatics

65. What is the cause of ARDS (adult respiratory distress syndrome)?

(A) excessive fluid administration
(B) pulmonary infection
(C) systemic sepsis
(D) The cause is unknown.

66. How is the PCWP (pulmonary capillary wedge pressure) used in the differentation of ARDS (adult respiratory distress syndrome) from cardiogenic-induced pulmonary edema?

(A) A low PCWP with large intrapulmonary shunts suggests ARDS.
(B) The PCWP rises in both ARDS and pulmonary edema but the PCWP in ARDS is usually over 30 mm Hg.
(C) The PCWP is low in ARDS but the CVP (central venous pressure) is elevated.
(D) The PCWP equals the CVP in ARDS but not pulmonary edema.

Questions 67 and 68 refer to the following scenario.

A 64-year-old female is admitted to your unit two days after CABG (coronary artery bypass graft) surgery. Symptoms include severe shortness of breath, which has developed over the past two hours; its cause is unknown. A chest x ray shows marked amounts of fluid in both lungs. Blood gas and pulmonary artery catheter information is as follows:

PULMONARY ARTERY CATHETER
blood pressure	98/64
pulse	114
PA	44/23
PCWP	12
CVP	3
CO	5.4
CI	2.9

BLOOD GASES
pH	7.35
$PaCO_2$	35
PaO_2	73
FIO_2	70%

67. Based on the preceding data, which condition is likely to be developing?

    (A) CHF (congestive heart failure)-induced pulmonary edema
    (B) sepsis from pulmonary infection
    (C) hypovolemia-induced left heart failure
    (D) ARDS (adult respiratory distress syndrome)

68. Which treatment is most likely indicated to support the preceding condition?

    (A) oxygen and PEEP (positive end expiratory pressure) therapy and fluid administration
    (B) oxygen and PEEP therapy and fluid restriction
    (C) mechanical ventilation and dobutamine
    (D) intubation, bicarbonate administration, and dopamine

69. Mortality with ARDS (adult respiratory distress syndrome) can be high, as much as 50%. What is the usual cause of death?

    (A) hypoxemia from the ARDS-induced intrapulmonary shunt
    (B) left ventricular failure induced by the ARDS
    (C) hypotension induced by the pulmonary capillary leak syndrome
    (D) the precipitating event that initiated the ARDS

Questions 70 and 71 refer to the following scenario.

A 74-year-old, 70-kg male is admitted to your unit with a diagnosis of respiratory failure secondary to pneumonia. He currently is intubated and on AMV (assisted mandatory ventilation), with a V_T of 750 cc, ventilator respiratory rate of 10, total rate of 29. His blood gas values are as follows:

pH	7.48
$PaCO_2$	30
PaO_2	64
FIO_2	80%

70. Based on the preceding information, which type of respiratory failure exists?

    (A) oxygenation failure
    (B) ventilation failure
    (C) combined oxygenation and ventilation failure
    (D) Neither oxygenation nor ventilation failure exists.

71. Which treatment would be indicated based on the blood gas values given?

(A) increase the ventilator V_T

(B) decrease the ventilator rate

(C) add PEEP (positive end expiratory pressure) therapy to reduce the FIO_2

(D) reduce the FIO_2 while increasing the ventilator peak flow rate

72. Which system gives more stable FIO_2 therapy?

(A) simple face mask

(B) nasal cannula

(C) rebreathing mask

(D) Venturi mask

73. At which level of FIO_2 support is oxygen toxicity thought to develop?

(A) 30 to 40% for longer than 48 hours

(B) 40 to 50% for longer than two hours

(C) >50% for longer than 24 hours

(D) FIO_2 does not cause oxygen toxicity; high PaO_2 values are the cause of toxicity.

74. Which of the following is an indication for PEEP (positive end expiratory pressure) therapy?

(A) to improve CO_2 elimination

(B) to treat a metabolic acidosis

(C) to reduce postoperative bleeding

(D) to allow reduction in FIO_2 levels

75. When PEEP (positive end expiratory pressure) or CPAP (continuous positive airway pressure) is used, which of the following values is monitored by the nurse to assess the effectiveness of therapy?

(A) mean arterial pressure

(B) right atrial pressure

(C) $PaCO_2$ levels

(D) SaO_2 values

76. Which of the following modes of ventilation is best for reducing the work of breathing?

(A) IRV (inverse ratio ventilation)
(B) IMV (intermittent mandatory ventilation)
(C) PSV (pressure support ventilation)
(D) AMV (assisted mandatory ventilation)

Questions 77 and 78 refer to the following scenario.

A 38-year-old female is admitted with respiratory failure secondary to viral pneumonitis. She is currently on AMV (assisted mandatory ventilation) with a ventilator rate of 12, total rate of 26, V_T of 800, FIO_2 of 80%, and peak airway pressures of 38. SpO_2 values are about 0.93. She suddenly becomes restless and indicates that she is short of breath. Her finger oximeter value decreases to 0.83. Breath sounds are diminished on the right with peak airway pressures of 52 cm H_2O.

77. Based on the preceding information, which condition is likely to be developing?

(A) ARDS (adult respiratory distress syndrome)
(B) pneumonia
(C) pneumothorax
(D) pericardial tamponade

78. Treatment would most likely include which of the following measures?

(A) administration of morphine and Lasix
(B) addition of 5 cm of PEEP (positive end expiratory pressure)
(C) administration of dobutamine
(D) insertion of a chest tube

79. PSV (pressure support ventilation) differs from IMV (intermittent mandatory ventilation) and AMV (assisted mandatory ventilation) in which of the following ways?

(A) PSV includes a level of PEEP (positive end expiratory pressure) with each breath.
(B) PSV is negative pressure regulated.
(C) IMV and AMV are volume limited, PSV pressure limited.
(D) IMV and AMV do not reduce the work of breathing, whereas PSV reduces the work of breathing and is therefore a better weaning tool.

80. Which of the following is an indication of potential ability to breathe spontaneously when removed from the ventilator?

(A) vital capacity of 5 cc/kg
(B) tidal volume of 1 to 2 cc/kg
(C) peak inspiratory pressures less than 20 cm H_2O
(D) minute ventilation of 5 to 10 LPM

Questions 81 and 82 refer to the following scenario.

A 58-year-old, 80-kg male is recovering from acute respiratory failure. He has been on mechanical ventilation for five days and was previously in good health. He currently has no shortness of breath and is on an IMV (intermittent mandatory ventilation) of 12 with a total respiratory rate of 18. His FIO_2 is 0.40 with a PaO_2 of 98, a $PaCO_2$ of 36, pH of 7.42. He has the following weaning parameters:

VT	410 cc
VC	950 cc
PIP	−29 cm H_2O
VE	9 LPM
respiratory rate	22

81. Based on the preceding information, which form of weaning is most likely to be implemented?

(A) IMV (intermittent mandatory ventilation)
(B) IRV (inverse ratio ventilation)
(C) T-piece trial
(D) PSV (pressure support ventilation)

Before answering question 82, read the following additional information.
    After one hour on a T-piece trial, the following additional information is available:

VT	450 cc
VC	950 cc
PIP	−38 cm H_2O
VE	8.3 LPM
respiratory rate	18
SaO_2	96%
PaO_2	85
$PaCO_2$	39
pH	7.39

82. Based on the additional information, what should be the next step in weaning this patient?

(A) Place him back on the ventilator and repeat the attempt later.
(B) Change to PSV (pressure support ventilation) weaning.
(C) Extubation is indicated.
(D) Rest one more day, then extubate.

Questions 83 through 85 refer to the following scenario.

A 63-year-old male is admitted with acute respiratory distress. Symptoms include marked shortness of breath and circumoral cyanosis. He is awake but is beginning to be less responsive. He has a history of COPD (chronic obstructive pulmonary disease). Blood gases reveal the following information:

pH	7.22
$PaCO_2$	62
PaO_2	54
SaO_2	0.81
HCO_3-	25
FIO_2	30%

83. Based on the preceding information, which condition is likely to be developing?

(A) CHF (congestive heart failure)
(B) ARDS (adult respiratory distress syndrome)
(C) acute respiratory failure
(D) pulmonary emboli

84. What would be the first treatment indicated at this time?

(A) increase the FIO_2
(B) intubate and place on mechanical ventilation
(C) postural drainage treatment
(D) aminophylline aerosol treatment

85. What is the cause of hypoxemia in this patient?

(A) diffusion barrier
(B) intrapulmonary shunt
(C) anatomic shunt
(D) hypoventilation

86. Which of the following is a complication of mechanical ventilation and PEEP (positive end expiratory pressure) therapy?

(A) atelectasis
(B) oxygen toxicity
(C) reduced cardiac output
(D) ARDS (adult respiratory distress syndrome)

87. What is the highest FIO_2 that can generally be achieved with a nasal cannula?

(A) 30%
(B) 40%
(C) 50%
(D) 100%

Questions 88 and 89 refer to the following scenario.

A 70-year-old male is in your unit with a diagnosis of exacerbation of COPD (chronic obstructive pulmonary disease), probably a pneumonia-induced event. He has very thick secretions, which have been difficult to remove during endotracheal suctioning.

88. Which of the following is the best method to aid in removal of thick secretions?

(A) instillation of saline
(B) increasing the suction pressure
(C) stimulation of his cough reflex
(D) increasing the humidity of his oxygen

89. Failure to remove the secretions will produce which effect on blood gases?

(A) decrease in $PaCO_2$
(B) decrease in PaO_2
(C) increase in pH
(D) increase in HCO_3- levels

90. What is the optimal level of PEEP (positive end expiratory pressure) therapy?

(A) the highest level of PEEP that increases cardiac output
(B) the highest level of PEEP that stabilizes $PaCO_2$ and PaO_2
(C) the lowest level of PEEP that improves cardiac output and SaO_2
(D) the lowest level of PEEP that increases the PaO_2 without depressing the cardiac output

91. Which of the following conditions produces the condition whose physical description is that of a "blue bloater"?

(A) emphysema
(B) asthma
(C) superior vena caval syndrome
(D) chronic bronchitis

92. Which of the following conditions produces the condition whose physical description is that of a "pink puffer"?

(A) emphysema
(B) asthma
(C) acute hyperventilation
(D) chronic bronchitis

93. Which of the following conditions is most likely to benefit from postural drainage and percussion?

(A) emphysema
(B) CHF (congestive heart failure)
(C) asthma
(D) chronic bronchitis

94. Which of the following conditions is associated with the greatest increase in work of breathing?

(A) emphysema
(B) bronchiectasis
(C) pneumonia
(D) chronic bronchitis

95. α_1-Antitrypsin deficiencies produce which type of condition?

(A) asthma
(B) emphysema
(C) bronchitis
(D) recurrent pneumonias

Questions 96 through 98 refer to the following scenario.

A 56-year-old male is admitted to your unit with acute shortness of breath. He has a 30-pack-per-year history of smoking. He has had no prior medical problems before this event, although he has noted exercise limitation over the past few years. On physical examination, he is slightly overweight, has jugular venous distension and has peripheral cyanosis. Blood gas studies reveal the following:

pH	7.35
$PaCO_2$	58
PaO_2	54
SaO_2	0.84
FIO_2	2 LPM via nasal cannula

96. Based on the preceding information, which condition is likely to be present?

(A) chronic bronchitis
(B) emphysema
(C) CHF (congestive heart failure)
(D) pulmonary emboli

97. What is your interpretation of the blood gas values?

(A) acute uncompensated respiratory acidosis
(B) acute uncompensated respiratory alkalosis
(C) compensated respiratory acidosis
(D) compensated metabolic acidosis

98. Which treatment would be most effective in this patient?

(A) intubation and mechanical ventilation
(B) CPAP (continuous positive airway pressure) therapy
(C) diuretics and digoxin
(D) oxygen therapy and bronchodilators

99. Which of the following is an example of the bronchodilator category of methylxanthines?

(A) terbutaline
(B) albuterol
(C) metaproterenol
(D) theophylline

100. Low PaO_2 levels produce at least three physiologic reactions. Which of the following is NOT a consequence of low PaO_2 levels?

(A) pulmonary hypertension
(B) increased drive to breathe
(C) low SaO_2 levels
(D) left shift of the oxyhemoglobin dissociation curve

101. If the finger oximeter is reading 0.97 and the PaO_2 is 63, what may we infer about the oxyhemoglobin dissociation curve?

(A) A left shift in the oxyhemoglobin dissociation curve exists.
(B) A right shift in the oxyhemoglobin dissociation curve exists.
(C) The oxyhemoglobin dissociation curve is in a normal position.
(D) The oxyhemoglobin dissociation curve cannot be correlated with SaO_2 and PaO_2 values.

102. If the oxyhemoglobin dissociation curve shifts to the right, what is the clinical implication?

(A) Oxygen is more readily dissociated from hemoglobin.
(B) Hemoglobin binds oxygen more tightly.
(C) Erythropoietin stimulation will increase hemoglobin levels.
(D) Phosphate levels will be depleted.

Questions 103 and 104 refer to the following scenario.

A 70-year-old female is admitted to your unit with the diagnosis of exacerbation of COPD (chronic obstructive pulmonary disease). She currently is short of breath, is using accessory muscles to breathe, and complains of difficulty eating over the past several weeks due to her shortness of breath. Her blood pressure is 142/88, pulse rate 108. She has the following laboratory information:

pH	7.39
$PaCO_2$	32
PaO_2	59
FIO_2	room air
hemoglobin	10

103. Based on the preceding information, which condition is likely to be present?

(A) chronic bronchitis
(B) emphysema
(C) asthma
(D) pulmonary emboli

104. Which of the following treatments would most improve her oxygen transport status?

(A) oxygen therapy
(B) blood transfusion
(C) CPAP (continuous positive airway pressure) therapy
(D) IPPB (intermittent positive pressure breathing) treatment

105. Assume that you want to reduce the FIO_2 of a patient after CABG (coronary artery bypass graft) surgery. No prior history of lung disease exists and his intrapulmonary shunt is near normal. How long is it necessary to wait to obtain blood gases or oximetry results after changing the FIO_2?

(A) 5 to 10 minutes
(B) 15 to 20 minutes
(C) 20 to 30 minutes
(D) 30 to 60 minutes

106. Which combination of treatments would be most effective in treating status asthmaticus?

(A) corticosteriods and bronchodilators
(B) methylxanthines and antibiotics
(C) postural drainage and bronchodilators
(D) oxygen and bronchodilators

Questions 107 through 109 refer to the following scenario.

A 24-year-old female is admitted to your unit in acute respiratory distress with the diagnosis of asthma. Lung auscultation reveals generalized wheezing. She is compliant with medications at home. She has received epinephrine and aminophylline in the emergency room with no improvement of her symptoms. Her blood gases reveal the following:

pH	7.48
$PaCO_2$	27
PaO_2	59
FIO_2	4 LPM via nasal cannula
HCO_3^-	23

107. Based on the preceding information, which condition is likely to be developing?

(A) pneumonia
(B) status asthmaticus
(C) pulmonary emboli
(D) ARDS (adult respiratory distress syndrome)

108. Assume the FIO_2 is increased to 6 LPM. Which of the following blood gas values would be an indication of a worsening status?

	(A)	(B)	(C)	(D)
pH	7.36	7.52	7.37	7.44
$PaCO_2$	30	24	37	29
PaO_2	70	64	72	59

109. Physical assessment by the nurse is one of the keys to evaluation of therapy. During auscultation of the patient's lungs, what should the nurse be aware of if a reduction in the degree of wheezing were to occur?

(A) Her condition may be worsening or improving.
(B) Reduction in wheezing always indicates improvement.
(C) Right ventricular failure is developing.
(D) Pulmonary hypertension is being alleviated.

110. What is the definition of status asthmaticus?

(A) the first episode of a newly diagnosed asthmatic
(B) the preterminal asthmatic episode
(C) an asthma episode that has failed to improve with conventional treatment
(D) an asthma episode that is complicated by CHF (congestive heart failure)

111. Pulmonary emboli produce all of the following physiologic changes but one. Which of the following is NOT likely to occur with pulmonary emboli?

(A) pulmonary hypertension
(B) arterial hypoxemia
(C) hypocarbia (low $PaCO_2$)
(D) congestive heart failure

112. Which of the following tests is most diagnostic for pulmonary emboli?

(A) blood gas analysis
(B) ventilation/perfusion scans
(C) pulmonary angiography
(D) pulmonary function tests

113. Effects from recurrent emboli due to deep venous thrombosis can be avoided by which one of the following therapies?

(A) use of a Greenfield (inferior vena caval) filter
(B) heparin
(C) coumadin
(D) use of lower extremity alternating compression devices

Questions 114 and 115 refer to the following scenario.

A 34-year-old female is admitted to your unit three weeks following cesarean delivery with acute shortness of breath and right chest pain. She has no prior cardiopulmonary medical history. She has the following blood gas values:

pH	7.46
$PaCO_2$	30
PaO_2	62
FIO_2	3 LPM

114. Based on the preceding information, which condition is likely to be developing?

   (A) ARDS (adult respiratory distress syndrome)
   (B) dissecting thoracic aneurysm
   (C) pleuritis
   (D) pulmonary emboli

115. Which treatment would most likely improve her immediate symptoms?

   (A) heparin
   (B) oxygen therapy
   (C) TPA (tissue plasminogen activator) or streptokinase
   (D) aminophylline

116. Which of the following features of pleural drainage systems indicates an active pleural leak?

   (A) bubbling in the water seal chamber
   (B) bubbling in the suction control chamber
   (C) fluctuation of water level in the water seal chamber with respiration
   (D) no fluctuation of water level in the water seal chamber with respiration

Questions 117 and 118 refer to the following scenario.

A 18-year-old male is admitted to your unit following thoracic trauma from a motor vehicle accident. He has a right chest tube in place. The chest tube has bubbling in both the water seal and suction control chambers. During transport to the radiology department, the chest drainage unit is broken when the transport cart is pushed against a wall. The chest tube is essentially open to air.

117. Based on the preceding information, which type of pneumothorax has most likely been created?

   (A) closed pneumothorax
   (B) open pneumothorax
   (C) tension pneumothorax
   (D) sealed pneumothorax

118. Which of the following would be the best treatment strategy?

(A) clamp the chest tube

(B) leave the tube open until a new unit is put in place

(C) leave the broken unit on temporarily but add suction to the suction control chamber

(D) place Vaseline gauze over the chest insertion site and clamp the chest tube

119. Which type of condition can lead to a tension pneumothorax?

(A) closed pneumothorax

(B) open pneumothorax

(C) subcutaneous emphysema

(D) pneumomediastinum

120. Which type of rib fracture has the highest complication rate?

(A) first rib

(B) third rib

(C) fifth rib

(D) seventh rib

Questions 121 and 122 refer to the following scenario.

A 42-year-old female is admitted to your unit following a motor vehicle accident. She has injuries to the sternum and neck. X rays in the emergency room reveal no obvious injuries. After one hour in the unit, she complains of sudden, severe shortness of breath. She is extremely anxious. On examination, you notice that she has developed subcutaneous emphysema across her chest. Her breath sounds are equal but markedly diminished. The trachea is midline.

121. Based on the preceding information, which condition is likely to be developing?

(A) tension pneumothorax

(B) tracheal laceration

(C) closed pneumothorax

(D) pneumomediastinum

122. Which treatment is indicated for this condition?

(A) immediate surgery

(B) chest tube insertion

(C) pericardiocentesis

(D) thoracocentesis

123. Which of the following findings would be an indication of a ruptured diaphram?

(A) diminished bowel sounds
(B) tracheal shift toward the affected diaphragm
(C) irregular breathing
(D) bowel sounds in the chest

124. An anterior chest tube for the drainage of the air causing a pneumothorax is usually placed in which ICS (intercostal space)?

(A) first ICS, anterior clavicular line
(B) second ICS, midclavicular line
(C) fourth ICS, anterior axillary line
(D) sixth ICS, midaxillary line

125. A posterior chest tube for the drainage of fluid from the pleural space is usually placed in which ICS (intercostal space)?

(A) second ICS, midclavicular line
(B) fourth ICS, anterior axillary line
(C) fifth ICS, midaxillary line
(D) seventh ICS, midaxillary line

Questions 126 and 127 refer to the following scenario.

A 26-year-old male is admitted to your unit from the emergency room with chest injuries following a motor vehicle accident. He complains of chest pain and shortness of breath. The right side of his chest [between the fourth and seventh ICSs (intercostal spaces)] moves in on inspiration and out on expiration. A chest x ray shows fractured ribs of the third through eighth ICSs.

126. Based on the preceding information, which condition is likely to be developing?

(A) tension pneumothorax
(B) hemopneumothorax
(C) pericardial tamponade
(D) flail chest

127. Which treatment would be best advised for this patient?

(A) open thoracotomy
(B) positive pressure ventilation
(C) external rib fixation with sandbags
(D) supportive therapy, such as oxygen therapy and pain relief

Questions 128 and 129 refer to the following scenario.

A 41-year-old female is admitted to your unit following a fall from the roof of her single-story house, having landed on her chest. She complains of chest pain; breath sounds are equal without diminished sound. Her trachea is midline, respirations indicate normal expansion of thorax. Her blood pressure is 130/88, pulse 122, respiratory rate 29. ECG (electrocardiogram) is within normal limits. Neck veins are not distended. Heart sounds reveal S_1, S_2 and soft S_3.

128. Based on the preceding information, which condition would need to be ruled out?

(A) cardiac rupture
(B) cardiac tamponade
(C) cardiac contusion
(D) pneumomediastinum

129. Which treatment would be indicated based on this scenario?

(A) cardiac surgery
(B) insertion of mediastinal chest tubes
(C) pericardiocentesis
(D) supportive, treating symptoms as they occur

130. Which of the following would best establish the diagnosis of cardiac contusion?

(A) Analysis of CPK-MB (creatine phosphokinase–CPK-MB) isoenzymes
(B) monitoring of heart sounds
(C) 12-lead ECG
(D) pulmonary artery (Swan-Ganz) catheterization

Questions 131 and 132 refer to the following scenario.

A 23-year-old female is admitted to your unit from the emergency room following a motor vehicle accident. She has no apparent injuries, although a chest x ray indicated a fourth-rib fracture on the left and a fifth-rib fracture on the right. Shortly after arrival in the unit, she develops marked shortness of breath and manifests a rightward deviation of the trachea and diminished breath sounds on the left. Her blood pressure is 94/62, pulse 120, respiratory rate 32.

131. Based on the preceding information, what condition is likely to be developing?

(A) open pneumothorax
(B) tension pneumothorax
(C) cardiac tamponade
(D) flail chest

132. What would be the best treatment for this condition?

(A) insertion of pleural chest tubes
(B) insertion of mediastinal chest tubes
(C) open thoracotomy
(D) pericardiocentesis

133. A 38-year-old male is admitted to your unit following a fall from a bicycle. He has sustained possible fractures of the sixth through ninth ribs on the right. Which of the following could be physical signs of fractured ribs without a pneumothorax?

  I. decreased breath sounds over the area
  II. shallow breathing
 III. splinting of the affected side

(A) I and II
(B) I and III
(C) II and III
(D) I, II, and III

134. In a patient admitted with the diagnosis of cardiac contusion, which physical sign would correlate best with this diagnosis?

(A) distended neck veins
(B) tachycardia disproportionate to injury
(C) shortness of breath
(D) ecchymotic area over the entire sternum

CHAPTER 3 _____

Neurology Practice Exam

1. Which meningeal layer lies closest to the brain?

   (A) pia mater
   (B) dura mater
   (C) arachnoid
   (D) subarachnoid

2. Which cerebral component is responsible for reabsorbing CSF (cerebro-spinal fluid)?

   (A) lateral ventricle
   (B) dura mater
   (C) arachnoid villi
   (D) subarachnoid cisterns

3. Which meningeal layer lies closest to the skull?

   (A) pia mater
   (B) dura mater
   (C) arachnoid
   (D) subarachnoid

4. Which structure separates the left and right cerebral hemispheres?

   (A) dura mater
   (B) subarachnoid space
   (C) fissure of Rolando
   (D) falx cerebri

5. Crossing of impulses between the two hemispheres is made possible by which structure?

(A) corpus callosum
(B) lateral ventricle
(C) postcentral gyrus
(D) falx cerebri

6. An injury to the temporal lobe would cause disturbances in which sensory component?

(A) sight
(B) hearing
(C) spatial orientation
(D) taste

7. A patient in your unit has suffered frontal head injuries from a motor vehicle accident. Which type of impairment may result from injury to the frontal lobe?

(A) loss of sensation
(B) loss of vision
(C) alterations in hearing
(D) alterations in personality

8. Maintenance of an awake and alert status is dependent on the proper functioning of which two cerebral structures?

(A) reticular activating system and both cerebral hemispheres
(B) parietal and occipital lobes
(C) pons and basal ganglia
(D) thalamus and hypothalamus

9. The thalamus is resposible for integrating all of the following body sensations except one. Which sense does the thalamus NOT integrate?

(A) smell
(B) sight
(C) hearing
(D) touch

10. Neurohumoral control of respiration is located in which structure?

(A) pons
(B) medulla
(C) reticular activating system
(D) basal ganglia

11. The primary function of the cerebellum includes which of the following?

(A) thought integration
(B) maintenance of personality characteristics
(C) sensory reception
(D) maintenance of equilibrium and muscle coordination

12. The lateral ventricles are connected to the third ventricle via which structure?

(A) cerebral aquaduct of Sylvius
(B) choroid plexus
(C) foramen of Monro
(D) foramen of Magendie

13. Obstruction of the foramen of Monro would produce which condition?

(A) ipsilateral dilation of the pupils
(B) hydrocephalus
(C) hemiparesis
(D) compression of the third cranial nerve

14. CSF (cerebrospinal fluid) is synthesized by which structure?

(A) corticospinal tract
(B) subarachnoid villi
(C) lateral ventricle
(D) choroid plexus

15. Which of the following corresponds most closely to the primary purpose of the CSF (cerebrospinal fluid)?

(A) transport of oxygen to the brain
(B) manufacture of neurotransmitters
(C) cushioning the brain and spinal column
(D) maintenance of cerebral perfusion pressures

16. Which area of the brain governs all motor functions?

(A) parietal lobe
(B) frontal lobe
(C) occipital lobe
(D) temporal lobe

17. The parietal lobe is responsible for which function?

    (A) temperature regulation
    (B) sensory integration
    (C) motor function
    (D) vision

18. Which artery is responsible for anterior circulation to the brain?

    (A) external carotid
    (B) internal carotid
    (C) basilar
    (D) vertebral

19. Adrenergic fibers of the sympathetic nervous system release which of the following neurotransmitters?

    (A) serotonin and dopamine
    (B) dopamine and acetycholine
    (C) epinephrine and norepinephrine
    (D) acetycholine and GABA (γ-aminobutyric acid)

20. Autoregulation of the cerebral circulatory system is most sensitive to changes in which of the following parameters?

    (A) mean arterial pressure
    (B) PaO_2
    (C) pH
    (D) glucose level

21. Which area of the brain is most sensitive to hypoxia?

    (A) brainstem
    (B) cerebral cortex
    (C) cerebellum
    (D) subarachnoid villi

22. Which statement most accurately describes the circle of Willis?

    (A) It is located in the cerebrum.
    (B) It helps provide adequate circulation through its anastomosis.
    (C) It is responsible for sleep and wakefulness.
    (D) It is part of the brainstem.

23. Hypothalmic disorders would be manifested by disturbances in which function?

(A) water balance and temperature control
(B) sensory processing
(C) vision
(D) sensory organization

24. The gray matter of the spinal cord represents which type of tissue?

(A) dendrite
(B) axon
(C) unmyelinated tissue
(D) myelinated tissue

25. How are the descending tracts within the spinal cord best described?

(A) columns
(B) funiculi
(C) sensory
(D) motor

Questions 26 and 27 refer to the following scenario.

A patient is admitted to the intensive care unit after sustaining a knife wound to the back. Assessment findings include loss of pain and temperature on the right side and loss of motor function on the left. Vital signs are stable and he is alert and oriented. No other injuries are noted.

26. Based on the preceding information, which type of neurologic syndrome is likely to be developing?

(A) central cord
(B) Brown-Séquard
(C) anterior cord
(D) Horner

27. Which type of treatment would be best advised for this syndrome?

(A) insertion of spinal rods
(B) spinal stabilization
(C) insertion of cervical halo rings
(D) administration of endogenous neurotransmitters

28. Which of the following is a necessary immediate assessment for a C3-4 injury?

(A) heart rate
(B) motor ability
(C) temperature
(D) respiration

29. Which vital sign changes (due to loss of sympathetic nervous stimulation) would occur after a spinal cord lesion above T-5?

(A) bradycardia and hypotension
(B) hyperthermia and tachycardia
(C) tachycardia and hypotension
(D) hypotension and bradycardia

30. Which symptoms are present in cases of autonomic hyperreflexia?

(A) bradycardia and hypertension
(B) hyperthermia and tachycardia
(C) tachycardia and hypotension
(D) hypertension and hyperthermia

31. The presence of a positive extensor plantar (Babinski) reflex in an unconscious patient indicates which situation?

(A) a lower motor neuron lesion
(B) an upper motor neuron lesion
(C) peripheral nerve damage
(D) an intact spinal arc

32. All of the following are symptoms of a basilar skull fracture but one. Which symptom is NOT indicative of a basilar skull fracture?

(A) rhinorrhea and otorrhea
(B) Battle sign, raccoon eyes
(C) tinnitus, nystagmus, and hearing difficulty
(D) loss of consciousness and dilated pupils

33. Which of the following corresponds most closely to the range of adequate cerebral perfusion pressures?

(A) >30 mm Hg
(B) <60 mm Hg
(C) >60 mm Hg
(D) any value less than the intracranial pressure

34. Which of the following can cause an epidural hematoma?

(A) skull fracture lacerating the middle meningeal artery
(B) rupture of an intracranial aneurysm
(C) infectious meningitis
(D) cerebral edema

35. Where are intracranial aneurysms most commonly found?

(A) external carotid arteries
(B) circle of Willis
(C) internal carotid arteries
(D) vertebral arteries

36. A 28-year-old male is admitted to the intensive care unit with a diagnosis of closed head injury. The nurse should be aware of which potential complications?

(A) hypotension
(B) respiratory alkalosis
(C) tremors
(D) cerebral edema

37. Hyperventilation, as a treatment modality for cerebral edema, should be maintained at which range for maximum effect?

(A) 25 to 30 mm Hg
(B) 35 to 40 mm Hg
(C) 40 to 45 mm Hg
(D) 50 to 55 mm Hg

38. Which of the following is a common cause of intracerebral hemorrhage?

(A) cerebral edema
(B) hypertensive encephalopathies
(C) prolonged hypotensive episodes
(D) Valsalva maneuvers

39. Cerebral perfusion pressure is calculated according to which of the following formulas?

(A) MAP (mean arterial pressure) – ICP (intracranial pressure)
(B) systolic blood pressure – ICP
(C) ICP + cerebral blood flow
(D) MAP + ICP

Questions 40 and 41 refer to the following scenario.

A 45-year-old male is admitted to your unit with a diagnosis of intracranial hypertension due to subarachnoid hemorrhage. The current vital signs include a blood pressure of 180/90, ICP (intracranial pressure) 15, pulse 140, respiratory rate 20.

40. Based on the preceding information, what is the cerebral perfusion pressure?

(A) 90
(B) 105
(C) 120
(D) It cannot be calculated.

41. Which of the following are measures that would improve the cerebral perfusion pressure?

   I. decrease the ICP (intracranial pressure)
   II. decrease the MAP (mean arterial pressure)
   III. decrease the heart rate
   (A) I
   (B) I and II
   (C) II and III
   (D) I, II, and III

42. Which of the following corresponds most closely to the range of minimum cerebral perfusion pressures?

(A) 30 to 40 mm Hg
(B) 40 to 50 mm Hg
(C) 50 to 60 mm Hg
(D) >60 mm Hg

43. What is an acceptable normal ICP (intracranial pressure)?

(A) −5 to +5 mm Hg
(B) 5 to 10 mm Hg
(C) 10 to 20 mm Hg
(D) >20 mm Hg

44. Nursing interventions for the patient with an ICP (intracranial pressure) monitoring device include which of the following?

(A) routine flushing of the system with heparinized saline
(B) maintaining the transducer at the level of the heart
(C) administration of prophylactic antibiotics
(D) monitoring the patient for signs and symptoms of infection

45. The hypothalamus secretes which hormone to regulate water balance?

(A) aldosterone
(B) renin
(C) ADH (antidiuretic hormone)
(D) oxytocin

46. Approximately two-thirds of the brain's blood supply is transported through which artery?

(A) internal carotid
(B) anterior communicating
(C) vertebral
(D) middle meningeal

47. What percent of total body oxygen consumption is accounted for by the brain?

(A) 2 to 5%
(B) 5 to 10%
(C) 10 to 15%
(D) >15%

48. How much of a reserve of oxygen exists in the brain?

(A) 100 cc
(B) 225 cc
(C) 450 cc
(D) No reserve exists.

49. Of the following factors, which does NOT play a role in maintaining consciousness?

(A) cerebral perfusion pressure
(B) oxygen transport level
(C) adequate blood glucose level
(D) normal serum potassium level

50. The reticular activating system is responsible for which of the following functions?

(A) motor control of skeletal muscle
(B) relay of sensory impulses to the parietal lobe
(C) sleep and wakefulness
(D) secretion of all neurotransmitters

Questions 51 and 52 refer to the following scenario.

A 56-year-old factory worker is admitted to your unit following a 20-foot fall from a scaffold. He is unresponsive on admission to the emergency room and is taken to the operating room for a craniotomy. Upon return to the intensive care unit, he has had an evacuation of an epidural hematoma from a depressed skull fracture. He has an ICP (intracranial pressure) monitor (subarachnoid screw) in place. During the first postoperative day, you note on the ICP waveform pressures of approximately 12 mm Hg. C waves are evident. His level of consciousness is variable, with a Glasgow Coma Score of 12 upon stimulation.

51. Based on the preceding information, which condition is likely to be developing?

    (A) increased ICP (intracranial pressure)
    (B) possible rebleeding, as indicated by the lack of an A wave presence
    (C) an obstruction of the catheter due to the presence of C waves
    (D) A normal postoperative situation exists.

52. Which treatment should be undertaken for this condition?

    (A) apply a closed CSF (cerebrospinal fluid) drainage system
    (B) increase the frequency of ICP (intracranial pressure) monitoring
    (C) flush the ICP catheter with normal saline
    (D) No treatment is necessary.

53. Neurogenic hyperventilation is associated with damage to which structure?

    (A) cerebral cortex
    (B) cerebellum
    (C) thalamus
    (D) brainstem

54. Initial assessment of the neurologically impaired patient should include measurement of which of the following?

    (A) level of consciousness
    (B) pupillary eye movement
    (C) deep tendon reflexes
    (D) brainstem reflexes

55. A fixed and dilated pupil indicates compression of which cranial nerve?

    (A) I
    (B) II
    (C) III
    (D) IV

Questions 56 through 58 refer to the following scenario.

A 79-year-old female is in the intensive care unit following a head injury from a fall down a series of steps. Currently she is unresponsive, opens her eyes with painful stimuli, withdraws to pain in a decerebrate manner, and makes groaning noises when she is given a painful stimulus. During your examination at the start of your shift, you notice that the left pupil is larger than the right, whereas previous examinations noted pupillary equality.

56. Based on the preceding information, what is the Glasgow Coma Score?

(A) 3
(B) 7
(C) 9
(D) 15

57. What does the change in pupillary size potentially indicate?

(A) decrease in cerebral perfusion pressure
(B) loss of upper motor neuron function
(C) loss of cerebellar function
(D) increased ICP (intracranial pressure)

58. Treatment for this condition could include which of the following measures?

(A) cervical support
(B) spinal tap to relieve increased ICP (intracranial pressure)
(C) mechanical ventilation to augment MAP (mean arterial pressure)
(D) osmotic diuretics

59. Which waveform is considered pathologic in monitoring ICP (intracranial pressure)?

(A) A wave
(B) B wave
(C) C wave
(D) D wave

60. Which structure(s) is/are a part of the supratentorial space?

(A) cerebellum
(B) pons
(C) cerebral hemispheres
(D) cranial nerves

61. Which of the following is a common complication of a ruptured intracranial aneurysm?

(A) hypotension due to hypovolemia
(B) cardiac dysrhythmias
(C) acid-base disturbances
(D) vasospasm of cerebral arteries

62. The risk of rebleeding after the initial rupture of an intracranial aneurysm is greatest during which time period?

(A) within the first three days after initial bleeding
(B) between the 7th and 11th days after initial bleeding
(C) after surgical clipping of the aneurysm
(D) within the first 24 hours after initial bleeding

63. Signs and symptoms of meningeal irritation include all of the following EXCEPT:

(A) nuchal rigidity and headache
(B) Kernig and Brudzinski signs
(C) aphasia and paresis
(D) photophobia

64. Which of the following is an early sign of central herniation syndrome?

(A) dilated pupils
(B) respiratory depression
(C) papilledema
(D) depressed level of consciousness

65. Which of the following are brainstem reflexes?

(A) pupillary light reflexes
(B) oculocephalic responses
(C) oculovestibular responses
(D) spinal reflexes

66. Decerebrate posturing is characterized by which of the following?

(A) abnormal extension response
(B) abnormal flexion response
(C) hyperflexion of the lower extremities
(D) absent motor response

67. Diagnostic procedures usually performed when intracranial hypertension is suspected may include all of the following but one. Which of the following procedures is NOT performed?

(A) CAT (computed axial tomographic) scan
(B) lumbar puncture
(C) ventriculostomy
(D) cranial nerve examination

68. Nursing interventions for the patient having seizures include all of the following EXCEPT:

(A) protecting the patient from injury
(B) observing seizure precautions
(C) administering anticonvulsive drugs such as dilantin
(D) restraining the patient

69. The nurse should be aware of the characteristics of psychomotor seizures. Which of the following statements regarding psychomotor seizures is true?

    (A) They are psychological in origin.
    (B) The patient usually becomes unconscious.
    (C) They involve repetitive behavioral patterns.
    (D) They involve acts of random violence.

70. The most important treatment for the patient in status epilepticus is:

    (A) maintenance of a patent airway
    (B) administration of Valium
    (C) administration of glucose
    (D) administration of phenytoin

71. Pathophysiologic consequences of status epilepticus include all of the following except one. Which of the following consequences is NOT associated with status epilepticus?

    (A) hypoxemia
    (B) hypoglycemia
    (C) hyperthermia
    (D) hypothermia

Questions 72 and 73 refer to the following scenario.

A 71-year-old female is admitted to your unit with a possible CVA (cerebrovascular accident). She is currently responsive to painful stimuli and has a Glasgow Coma Score of 8. Her blood pressure is 180/110, pulse 64, respiratory rate 12. Her pupils are equal and reactive. During your shift, you note that her level of consciousness suddenly decreases. Upon examining her eyes, you note that the left pupil is large and unreactive to light. Vital signs are blood pressure 192/114, pulse 56, respiratory rate 10. Blood glucose level is 70.

72. Based on the preceding information, what has most likely occurred?

    (A) Decreasing ICP (intracranial pressure) has caused negative-pressure dysfunction of the second (optic) cranial nerve.
    (B) Hypoglycemia has occured.
    (C) Increasing MAP (mean arterial pressure) has decreased cerebral perfusion.
    (D) Increasing ICP has compressed the third (oculomotor) cranial nerve.

73. What is the prognostic implication of these physical changes?

(A) With aggressive treatment, neurologic function can be recovered.
(B) Neurologic function is unlikely to be recovered.
(C) Visual defects are likely to be permanent but other neurologic functions will recover.
(D) No implications regarding neurologic recovery can be drawn.

74. Myasthenia gravis is characterized by which of the following?

(A) ascending paralysis
(B) neuromuscular weakness with exercise and improvement with rest
(C) uncoordinated motor control
(D) peripheral sensory deficits

75. Which of the following is the major objective of therapy in myasthenia gravis?

(A) stimulate synaptic terminals to produce ACTH (adrenocorticotropic hormone)
(B) supportive care for the patient; the disease is self-limiting
(C) administration of anticholinesterase medications
(D) administration of ACTH

Questions 76 and 77 refer to the following scenario.

A 56-year-old male is admitted to your unit with a decreasing level of consciousness. His primary diagnosis is adenocarcinoma of the lung with possible metastatic spread to the brain. The family wants "everything done," which is why he has been admitted to the unit. His pupils are small but reactive. Respiration is cyclic, increasing in depth and rate and then characterized by short periods of apnea. Later in your shift, the level of consciousness decreases further, the pupils become dilated (3 to 4 mm) and unresponsive to light, and respiration increases in frequency and depth.

76. Based on the preceding information, which condition is likely to be developing?

(A) central herniation syndrome
(B) uncal herniation syndrome
(C) unilateral hemispheric compression
(D) pontine angle compression

77. Which of the following treatments would NOT be indicated in this situation?

(A) hyperventilation via mechanical ventilation
(B) osmotic diuretics
(C) corticosteroids
(D) spinal tap

78. Nursing interventions for myasthenia gravis include all of the following EXCEPT:

(A) monitoring ventilation status due to muscle weakness
(B) administration of aminoglycosides
(C) administration of anticholinesterase medications
(D) timing activities to avoid fatigue

79. Cholinergic crisis in myasthenia gravis is due to which of the following events?

(A) insufficient dose of medication
(B) overdose of medication
(C) fatigue, stress, or infection
(D) worsening of the disease process

80. Guillain-Barré syndrome affects which neurologic component?

(A) peripheral nervous system
(B) central nervous system
(C) autonomic nervous system
(D) Schwann cells

Questions 81 and 82 refer to the following scenario.

A patient of yours has been in a motor vehicle accident and has received cervical and spinal stabilization. He is alert and oriented with no evidence of head injury. He develops lower extremity paralysis on the same side as the wound and loses pain and temperature sensation on the side opposite the injury.

81. Based on the preceding information, this type of spinal injury response would be referred to as:

(A) total transection
(B) anterior cord syndrome
(C) central cord syndrome
(D) Brown-Séquard syndrome

82. Treatment for this condition would most likely include:

    (A) spinal tap for decompression
    (B) laminectomy
    (C) spinal traction
    (D) spinal fusion

83. A patient is admitted to the intensive care unit with signs and symptoms of ascending paralysis and respiratory failure. The critical care nurse would investigate for a past history of:

    (A) trauma to the spinal cord
    (B) trauma to the head
    (C) postviral, respiratory, or gastrointestinal infection
    (D) aspiration

84. Which of the following organisms is the most common cause of bacterial meningitis in adults?

    (A) *Meningococcus*
    (B) *Hemophilus influenzae*
    (C) *Staphylococcus*
    (D) *Pneumonococcus*

85. Clinical signs and symptoms of meningitis include all of the following EXCEPT:

    (A) positive Kernig and Brudzinki signs
    (B) headache and photophobia
    (C) hemiparesis and atrophy of muscles
    (D) photophobia and seizures

86. Which of the following are treatments for myasthenia gravis?

    I. pyridostigmine (Mestinon)
    II. neostigmine (Prostigmin)
    III. prednisone
        (A) I and II
        (B) II and III
        (C) I and III
        (D) I, II, and III

87. Which of the following surgical treatments may be useful in myasthenia gravis?

    (A) splenectomy
    (B) thymectomy
    (C) nerve transplants
    (D) pineal transplants

88. What is the reason that even a nonmalignant brain tumor may have dangerous consequences?

(A) Nonmalignant brain tumors can convert into malignant tumors.
(B) Brain tumors can secrete exogenous catecholamines.
(C) The mass in the brain can distort the ability to sense normal balance.
(D) Any mass will increase the ICP (intracranial pressure) due to the cranial structure's lack of distensibility.

89. Which of the following is NOT considered a neurotransmitter?

(A) dopamine
(B) dobutamine
(C) acetylcholine
(D) norepinephrine

90. Which of the following is the precursor to both epinephrine and norepinephrine?

(A) dopamine
(B) dobutamine
(C) acetylcholine
(D) norepinephrine

91. Which substrate does the brain depend most heavily upon for nutritional needs?

(A) fats
(B) proteins
(C) carbohydrates
(D) neurotransmitters

92. Anterior gray columns in the spinal cord contain cell bodies of which fiber type?

(A) afferent (sensory)
(B) efferent (motor)
(C) parasympathetic
(D) sympathetic synaptic

93. Fracture of which vertebra is termed the "hangman's fracture" due to the loss of spinal stabilization of the head?

(A) C-1
(B) C-3
(C) C-7
(D) T-1

94. Lesions of lower motor neurons cause which type of response?

(A) spastic muscle activity
(B) changes in level of consciousness
(C) changes in behavior
(D) flaccid paralysis

95. Lesions of upper motor neurons cause which type of response?

(A) spastic muscle activity
(B) changes in level of consciousness
(C) changes in behavior
(D) flaccid paralysis

Questions 96 and 97 refer to the following scenario.

A 19-year-old male is admitted to your unit following a motor vehicle accident. He currently is responsive but has no sensation below the upper chest area. Lateral cervical films reveal a possible C-6 fracture. A CAT scan reveals transection of the cord at C-6.

96. Based on the preceding information, what is the likelihood of the patient's recovering the ability to walk?

(A) good likelihood with rehabilitation
(B) good likelihood with surgery
(C) possible only if stabilization of the injury allows new spinal growth
(D) unlikely

97. Treatment of this condition would most likely include which of the following measures?

(A) supportive care since no treatment is effective
(B) surgical decompression
(C) bed rest on a spinal board
(D) cervical traction

98. Which condition characterizes upper and lower extremity weakness with more pronounced upper extremity weakness?

(A) Guillain-Barré syndrome
(B) Brown-Séquard syndrome
(C) central cord syndrome
(D) anterior cord syndrome

Questions 99 through 100 refer to the following scenario.

A 39-year-old construction worker is admitted to your unit after being crushed between two metal sheets. No head injury occurred and he is alert and oriented. He is able to sense pain and touch although the sensations are faint. He has no ability to move his legs or abdomen.

99. Based on the preceding information, which condition is likely to be present?

   (A) C-6 transection
   (B) Brown-Séquard syndrome
   (C) central cord syndrome
   (D) anterior cord syndrome

100. Which treatment would most likely be indicated for this condition?

   (A) supportive care since no treatment is effective
   (B) surgical decompression
   (C) bed rest on a spinal board
   (D) cervical traction

101. A patient sustains a spinal cord injury at C-6. He is conscious and alert. Barring complications, he should be able to perform all of the following actions EXCEPT one. Which action will he have difficulty performing?

   (A) diaphagmatic breathing
   (B) picking up objects with his fingers
   (C) reaching forward
   (D) sitting upright with support

102. A patient with cerebrospinal rhinorrhea would benefit most from which of the following?

   (A) assistance with nasal packing to tamponade the leak
   (B) insertion of a nasogastric tube to aspirate swallowed CSF (cerebrospinal fluid)
   (C) testing the CSF with litmus paper to determine the origin of the fluid
   (D) administration of prophylactic antibiotics

103. Which of the following is an example of a pure upper motor neuron lesion?

   (A) poliomyelitis
   (B) spinal cord injury below the level of L-1
   (C) amyotrophic lateral sclerosis
   (D) cerebrovascular accident with spastic paralysis

104. Which reflex is indicative of an upper motor neuron lesion?

(A) spinal reflex
(B) extensor plantar (Babinski) reflex
(C) anal wink
(D) Hering-Breuer reflex

105. A normal consensual light reflex indicates proper functioning of which two cranial nerves?

(A) abducens and acoustic
(B) ophthalmic and hypoglossal
(C) optic and oculomotor
(D) trochlear and vagal

106. What is the highest score on the Glasgow Coma Scale?

(A) 3
(B) 8
(C) 15
(D) 18

107. Which of the following would NOT cause a decrease in level of consciousness?

(A) right-sided cerebral infarct without cerebral edema
(B) glucose level less than 30
(C) cerebral perfusion pressure of 40
(D) oxygen transport of 400 cc/min

108. Given the following information, what is the cerebral perfusion pressure in this patient?

blood pressure	90/60
ICP	15
CVP	12
$PaCO_2$	35
PaO_2	88
pH	7.34

(A) 15
(B) 35
(C) 55
(D) 75

109. Which of the following would be least likely to produce a decreased level of consciousness?

(A) acute blunt head trauma
(B) acute CVA (cerebrovascular accident)
(C) old CVA
(D) diminished cerebral perfusion pressure

Questions 110 and 111 refer to the following scenario.

A 42-year-old female is in the unit following an assault. She suffered head lacerations although her CAT scan revealed no cerebral major injuries. She also received several stab wounds to the chest. The chest wounds have been treated but she remains hypoexemic. She has the following parameters:

blood pressure	100/70
pulse	90
CO	5 LPM
PCWP	12 mm Hg
CVP	5 mm Hg
PaO_2	50
FIO_2	0.70

The physician decides to add PEEP (positive end expiratory pressure) to this therapy in order to address the hypoxemia. Following are the new parameters:

blood pressure	90/60
pulse	110
CO	4 LPM
PCWP	13
CVP	15
PaO_2	98
FIO_2	0.70
PEEP	10

110. Based on the preceding information, what is your assessment of the change in oxygenation to the brain based on the addition of the PEEP?

(A) Oxygenation is worse based on the loss of cerebral perfusion pressure.
(B) Oxygenation is better based on improved PaO_2 and little change in cerebral perfusion.
(C) Oxygenation is unaffected since the ICP (intracranial pressure) is unchanged.
(D) Oxygenation cannot be approximated from these parameters.

111. What should be done from a treatment point of view based on the preceding information?

(A) No adjustment in treatment is necessary.
(B) Increase the PEEP to 12 cm as long as the ICP (intracranial pressure) is unchanged.
(C) Reduce the PEEP based on cerebral perfusion pressure.
(D) Administer a blood transfusion to improve oxygen transport.

112. Assume that a patient has a severe head injury and does not respond to verbal stimuli. Which of the following explains why asking the patient to squeeze your hand is not a good assessment tool?

(A) The auditory cranial nerve is likely to be damaged.
(B) Motor responses of the arm may be impaired.
(C) He may not understand your request.
(D) Latent primitive reflexes become operational with loss of higher cognitive function.

113. Impending central herniation is indicated by which of the following?

(A) decreased level of consciousness
(B) positive doll's eyes
(C) unilateral pupil dilation
(D) bilateral pupil dilation

114. Which of the following are signs of increasing ICP (intracranial pressure)?

(A) bradycardia and hypertension
(B) bradycardia and hypotension
(C) tachycardia and hypertension
(D) tachycardia and hypotension

115. Which of the following best describes the abnormal doll's eyes response?

(A) movement of the eyes in opposition to the movement of the head
(B) disconjugate eye movements
(C) movement of the eyes in the same direction as movement of the head
(D) eyes remaining stationary, midline, midposition

Questions 116 and 117 refer to the following scenario.

A patient is admitted after a motor vehicle accident with head and chest trauma. He requires a craniotomy with the insertion of an ICP (intracranial pressure) monitor. On the second postoperative day, he is responsive to stimuli and follows commands. Later in your shift, he becomes responsive only to painful stimuli. The following information is available:

blood pressure	90/58
pulse	107
ICP	24
CVP	13
serum glucose	92
PaO_2	68
$PaCO_2$	36

116. Based on the preceding information, what is the likely reason for the loss of responsiveness?

   (A) decreased substrate (i.e., glucose) availability
   (B) decreased PaO_2 levels
   (C) reduced ICP (intracranial pressure)
   (D) decreased cerebral perfusion pressure

117. Which structure primarily regulates the autonomic nervous system?

   (A) cerebellum
   (B) thalamus
   (C) hypothalamus
   (D) frontal lobe of the cerebral cortex

118. Which function is primarily regulated by the cerebellum?

   (A) speech
   (B) vision
   (C) coordination
   (D) respiration

119. Meningeal irritation is indicated by which of the following signs?

   (A) nuchal rigidity
   (B) Homans sign
   (C) positive extensor plantar (Babinski) reflex
   (D) flaccid paralysis

Questions 120 and 121 refer to the following scenario.

A 72-year-old female is admitted to the unit following a fall at home. Her daughter explains that her mother attempted to stand after dinner and immediately fell. Currently she is awake but unable to move her left side. She is able to talk and is alert and oriented. Admission vital signs are as follows:

blood pressure	176/110
pulse	62
respiratory rate	16
temperature	36.8° C

Pupils are equal and reactive; eye movements are normal. The patient states that she has been healthy and has never needed to "see a doctor."

120. Based on the preceding information, which condition is likely to be developing?

(A) left-sided CVA (cerebrovascular accident)
(B) internal carotid vasospasm
(C) right-sided CVA
(D) external carotid obstruction

121. Which neurologic test would be most helpful in establishing the diagnosis in this patient?

(A) CAT scan
(B) cold water caloric test
(C) oculocephalic testing
(D) EEG (electroencephalogram)

122. Which neurotransmitter is most important for synaptic transmission?

(A) serotonin
(B) acetylcholine
(C) dobutamine
(D) glucose

123. Contracoup head injuries manifest from which of the following mechanisms?

(A) injury to the side opposite the trauma
(B) injury to the side of the trauma
(C) cranial vault fracture due to high torque forces
(D) epidural tears from superficial scalp pressures

Questions 124 and 125 refer to the following scenario.

A 24-year-old female is admitted to your unit following a fall from a horse. After the fall, the horse kicked her in the temporal region of the head. She is admitted to the unit directly from the emergency room. She is unresponsive except to deep, painful stimuli. Head CAT scans reveal a temporal skull fracture. The following data are available:

blood pressure	84/52
pulse	112
respiratory rate	10

124. Based on the preceding information, which condition is likely to be developing?

(A) epidural hematoma
(B) subdural hematoma
(C) obstructive hydrocephalus
(D) contracoup head injury

125. Which treatment would be indicated based on the preceding data?

(A) increasing the ventilator rate
(B) placement of an ICP (intracranial pressure) monitor
(C) immediate craniotomy
(D) mannitol infusion

126. Which of the following is an indication of a basilar skull fracture?

(A) raccoon eyes
(B) decreasing pulse pressure
(C) spastic paralysis
(D) flaccid paralysis

127. Which of the following is the best description for Battle sign?

(A) generalized petechial development
(B) bleeding from the paranasal sinus
(C) hyperreflexia
(D) ecchymosis over the mastoid projection

128. Which type of head injury typically produces rapid clinical deterioration?

(A) subdural hematoma
(B) depressed skull fracture without displacement
(C) epidural hematoma
(D) subarachnoid hematoma

129. Which test is the most diagnostic for identifying head injuries?

(A) cranial x-rays
(B) lumbar puncture
(C) CAT scan
(D) PET (positron emission tomographic) scan

Questions 130 and 131 refer to the following scenario.

An 81-year-old male in your unit has a cerebral mass that has compressed the right optic tract. He is alert and oriented with no complaints except for visual disturbances. The physician has described the visual defect as left homonymous hemianopsia.

130. Which visual symptoms would be seen with this lesion?

(A) loss of vision in the right eye
(B) loss of vision in the left eye
(C) loss of periperal vision on the left and central vision on the right
(D) loss of peripheral vision on the right and central vision on the left

131. What should the nurse do with regard to placing items that might be needed by the patient?

(A) Instruct the patient not to reach for any items without assistance.
(B) No precautions are needed.
(C) Keep objects toward the right.
(D) Keep objects toward the left.

132. Myasthenia gravis is thought to occur due to which mechanism?

(A) loss of myelinated tissue
(B) disturbances in the reticular activating system
(C) deficient production of phenylephrine
(D) disturbance of acetylcholine utilization

Questions 133 and 134 refer to the following scenario.

A 37-year-old female is admitted to your unit with possible aspiration pneumonia. She has complained of a gradual increase in difficulty swallowing, which she believes is what precipitated her respiratory difficulties. During the examination, you note that she has ptosis of both eyes and has weak eye closure strength. Muscle weakness is generalized. No sensory deficits exist. She states that she fatigues easily although she recovers some strength after rest.

133. Based on the preceding information, which condition could be developing?

(A) multiple sclerosis
(B) Guillain-Barré syndrome
(C) Temporal lobe tumor
(D) myasthenia gravis

134. Which test would be performed to help identify the disease?

(A) administration of edrophonium chloride (Tensilon)
(B) six-minute walk
(C) administration of epinephrine
(D) CAT scan

135. Which of the following is NOT a treatment for myasthenia gravis?

(A) thymectomy
(B) Mestinon
(C) plasmapheresis
(D) Neosynephrine

136. A 69-year-old male has a cardiopulmonary arrest on the floor and is brought to your unit. Which of the following medications, if given previously, would interfere with an assessment of pupillary response?

I. atropine
II. epinephrine
III. lidocaine

(A) I
(B) I and II
(C) II and III
(D) I, II, and III

Questions 137 and 138 refer to the following scenario.

A 43-year-old male is admitted to your unit with complaints of severe headache, pain in the neck on flexion, and light sensitivity. He has no specific muscle weakness or sensory deficits. He has a positive Kernig sign. Vital signs are as follows:

blood pressure	142/84
pulse	118
respiratory rate	30
temperature	40° C

137. Based on the preceding information, which condition is likely to be developing?

(A) meningitis
(B) intracerebral bleeding
(C) myasthenia gravis
(D) subarachnoid bleeding

138. Which treatment would most likely be instituted?

(A) craniotomy
(B) administration of anticholinesterase agents
(C) insertion of a ventricular drain to reduce the increased ICP (intracranial pressure)
(D) administration of antibiotics

Questions 139 and 140 refer to the following scenario.

A 36-year-old male is admitted to your unit with rapidly increasing symptoms of generalized weakness following an episode of "flu." He noticed that the weakness started in his arms and legs and has progressed to his upper legs, abdomen, and chest. He has difficulty taking a deep breath. Vital signs are normal and he has some complaints of shortness of breath.

139. Based on the preceding symptoms, which condition is likely to be developing?

    (A) Guillain-Barré syndrome
    (B) myasthenia gravis
    (C) multiple sclerosis
    (D) amyotrophic lateral sclerosis

140. Which treatment is likely to be administered for this condition?

    (A) administration of anticholinesterase agents
    (B) supportive treatments, particularly of the respiratory system
    (C) administration of antibiotics
    (D) administration of sympathetic stimulation agents, such as norepinephrine

141. Which of the following best describes the Kernig sign?

    (A) muscle spasms in the arm upon occlusion with a blood pressure cuff
    (B) twitching of the face upon tapping the cheek
    (C) inability to flex the neck
    (D) inability to extend the leg when the thigh is flexed to the abdomen

142. The Brudzinski sign is best described by which of the following definitions?

    (A) adduction and flexion of the legs with neck flexion
    (B) pain in the neck upon raising the arms above shoulder level
    (C) temporary flaccid paralysis after neck compression
    (D) development of superficial muscle tremors after repetitive reflex testing

143. If a patient develops a grand mal (tonic-clonic) seizure, which initial nursing action should take place?

    (A) forcing an airway into the mouth
    (B) protecting the patient from injury
    (C) starting oxygen therapy
    (D) placing a padded tongue blade into the mouth

144. Which type of seizure starts in a localized manner and can develop into a grand mal seizure?

(A) focal (Jacksonian) motor seizure
(B) petit mal seizure
(C) akinetic seizure
(D) bilateral myoclonus (myoclonic seizure)

145. Which of the following is NOT a treatment for seizures?

(A) phenytoin sodium (Dilantin)
(B) phenobarbital
(C) diazepam (Valium)
(D) pancuronium bromide (Pavulon)

146. Status epilepticus is primarily dangerous for which of the following reasons?

(A) loss of cerebral oxygenation
(B) respiratory distress
(C) hemodynamic deterioration
(D) development of skeletal muscle damage

147. Which is the most common cause of a CVA (cerebrovascular accident)?

(A) cerebral bleeding
(B) thrombus formation
(C) coagulation defects
(D) excessive cerebral oxygen consumption

148. Which of the following is usually NOT considered an effective treatment for an acute CVA (cerebrovascular accident)?

(A) embolectomy
(B) craniotomy
(C) supportive measures
(D) administration of anticoagulants

149. Which of the following comprises most of the mass within the cranial vault?

(A) brain tissue
(B) intravascular volume
(C) CSF (cerebrospinal fluid)
(D) cerebral lining

150. Which of the following is NOT a compensating mechanism to offset or prevent a rise in ICP (intracranial pressure)?

(A) increasing MAP (mean arterial pressure) to overcome a rising ICP
(B) displacement of CSF (cerebrospinal fluid) from the brain to avoid increasing the ICP
(C) displacement of intravascular volume from the brain to avoid increasing the ICP
(D) displacement of brain tissue from the cranial vault to avoid increasing the ICP

CHAPTER 4 ———————————————

Gastroenterology Practice Exam

1. Secretion from the salivary glands is primarily regulated by which of the following?

   (A) central nervous system
   (B) autonomic nervous system
   (C) pituitary gland
   (D) hypothalamus

2. Atropine, a parasympathetic inhibitor, would cause which of the following physical symptoms due to parasympathetic action?

   (A) decreased salivary flow
   (B) increased level of consciousness
   (C) increased heart rate
   (D) decreased respiratory rate

3. Achalasia refers to which of the following?

   (A) decreased production of trypsin
   (B) increased backflow of gastric acid into the duodenum
   (C) loss of peristaltic waves in the small intestine
   (D) failure of the gastroesophageal sphincter

4. In which part of the gastrointestinal tract are no enzymes secreted?

   (A) mouth
   (B) esophagus
   (C) stomach
   (D) small intestine

Questions 5 and 6 refer to the following scenario.

A 26-year-old male is admitted to your unit complaining of chest pain unrelated to exercise. The pain is not relieved by rest. No ECG (electrocardiographic) changes are evident. The abdomen is soft and free from pain on palpation. Diet has been normal and no change in stool patterns has been reported. No problems with swallowing have been noted.

5. Based on the preceding information, what is the likely origin of the problem?

   (A) malfunction of the cardiac sphincter
   (B) duodenal ulcer
   (C) pyloric sphinchter reflux
   (D) myocardial ischemia

6. What treatment would most likely be instituted in this situation?

   (A) esophageal resection via the thoracic approach
   (B) antrectomy
   (C) vagotomy
   (D) diet change

7. Total gastrectomy would cause the patient to lose which function?

   (A) ability to secrete glucagon
   (B) bile production
   (C) vitamin B_{12} synthesis
   (D) acid-base regulation of chloride and bicarbonate

8. A 44-year-old male has a gastrostomy tube (G tube) placed for nutritional support following diagnosis of a malabsorptive syndrome. He is discharged with the G tube in place. Several weeks later, he is admitted to your unit with complaints of disorientation. The family states that they have been irrigating and aspirating the G tube following tube feedings. This irrigation of the G tube would most likely cause which disturbance?

   (A) metabolic acidosis
   (B) metabolic alkalosis
   (C) respiratory alkalosis
   (D) respiratory acidosis

9. Which substance will increase the production of hydrochloric acid?

   (A) histamine
   (B) atropine
   (C) bicarbonate
   (D) potassium salts

10. Cimetidine or ranitidine acts to reduce stress ulcers by inhibiting the production of which substance?

   (A) histamine
   (B) gastrin
   (C) acetylcholine
   (D) calcium

11. What is the purpose of the intrinsic factor, produced by parietal cells in the stomach?

   (A) promotes absorption of vitamin K
   (B) promotes absorption of vitamin B_{12}
   (C) increases utilization of vitamin C
   (D) synthesizes vitamin D with calcium

12. The normal pH of the stomach falls within which of the following ranges?

   (A) 1 to 3
   (B) 4 to 6
   (C) 6 to 8
   (D) >8

13. In which part of the gastrointestinal system is pepsinogen initially produced?

   (A) mouth
   (B) esophagus
   (C) stomach
   (D) small intestine

14. Which of the following is the most accurate definition of chyme?

   (A) a lipoprotein secreted in the stomach that aids in fat digestion
   (B) gastric cells responsible for negating excessive hydrochloric acid secretion
   (C) a hormone necessary for reducing the desire to eat
   (D) a semiliquid mass of food

15. Gastrin secretion causes which of the following effects?

   (A) increased desire to eat
   (B) inhibited desire to eat
   (C) production of vitamin B_{12}
   (D) increased production of hydrochloric acid

16. Which of the following is a function of cholecystokinin?

    (A) breaks down protein
    (B) inhibits gastric emptying
    (C) stimulates duodenal catabolism of carbohydrates
    (D) inhibits gallbladder activity

17. A vagotomy, through the removal of parasympathetic stimulation, can reduce hydrochloric acid secretion by which of the following mechanisms?

    (A) elimination of the cephalic phase of gastric secretion
    (B) elimination of the gastric phase of gastric secretion
    (C) elimination of the intestinal phase of gastric secretion
    (D) altering the ability of the stomach to sense the presence of food

18. Which of the following substrates is most readily processed by the gastrointestinal system?

    (A) fats
    (B) proteins
    (C) carbohydrates
    (D) lipoproteins

19. Approximately how many calories are in a gram of glucose?

    (A) 2 kcal
    (B) 4 kcal
    (C) 6 kcal
    (D) 9 kcal

20. Approximately how many calories are in a gram of fat?

    (A) 2 kcal
    (B) 4 kcal
    (C) 6 kcal
    (D) 9 kcal

21. Approximately how many calories are in a gram of protein?

    (A) 2 kcal
    (B) 4 kcal
    (C) 6 kcal
    (D) 9 kcal

22. D_5W has five grams of glucose per 100 cc of solution. Approximately how many calories are in one liter of D_5W?

(A) 20 kcal
(B) 200 kcal
(C) 500 kcal
(D) 2000 kcal

23. Which of the following enzymes is active in the digestion of proteins?

(A) amylase
(B) maltose
(C) lipase
(D) trypsin

24. Which of the following enzymes is active in the digestion of fats?

(A) amylase
(B) maltose
(C) lipase
(D) trypsin

25. Which of the following enzymes is active in the digestion of carbohydrates?

(A) amylase
(B) pepsin
(C) lipase
(D) trypsin

26. Emulsification (dispersion into small droplets) of fat occurs due to which substance?

(A) chyme
(B) lipase
(C) bile
(D) cholecystokinin

27. Following a gunshot wound to the abdomen, a 27-year-old male has a complete colectomy with creation of an ileostomy. What nursing measures will be necessary considering the fact that the function of the large intestine has been eliminated?

   I. administration of proteolytic enzymes via tube feedings
  II. observation of intake and output since reabsorption of water will be diminished
III. administration of emulsifying agents

    (A) I
    (B) II
    (C) I and III
    (D) II and III

28. What is the primary function of the small intestine?

(A) absorption of nutrients
(B) reabsorption of water
(C) reabsorption of carbon dioxide
(D) acting as a reservoir for food

29. Increased colonic motility is produced by which of the following?

(A) parasympathetic stimulation
(B) sympathetic stimulation
(C) central nervous system stimulation
(D) increased fat content in the diet

30. Which drug would potentially decrease colonic motility?

(A) nifedipine
(B) atropine
(C) digitalis
(D) gentamycin

31. All venous blood from the intestines eventually drains into which vein?

(A) gastric
(B) superior mesenteric
(C) portal
(D) celiac

32. The portal vein empties into which structure?

(A) inferior vena cava
(B) liver
(C) large intestine
(D) bile duct

33. Parasympathetic regulation of the gastrointestinal system is provided by which nerve?

(A) portal
(B) phrenic
(C) hepatic
(D) vagus

34. The sympathetic neurotransmitter norepinephrine is opposed by which parasympathetic neurotransmitter when regulating gastrointestinal activity?

(A) epinephrine
(B) dopamine
(C) serotonin
(D) acetylcholine

35. Which of the following is NOT a function of the pancreas?

(A) secretion of glucagon
(B) secretion of insulin
(C) secretion of potassium salts
(D) secretion of digestive enzymes

36. Which of the following enzymes is NOT secreted by the pancreas?

(A) pepsinogen
(B) trypsin
(C) lipase
(D) amylase

37. A duodenal feeding tube was placed by the RN on a prior shift. You want to check the placement of the tube in order to confirm that it is in the duodenum rather than the stomach. To check its position, you utilize a pH reading from aspirated tube contents. Which pH range would suggest a duodenal rather than a gastric location?

(A) 1 to 3
(B) 4 to 6
(C) 6 to 8
(D) >8

38. What is the function of hepatic Kupffer cells?

(A) phagocytosis
(B) production of pancreatic lipase
(C) production of bile
(D) stimulation of the microenzyme oxidizing system

39. Which of the following are major functions of the liver?

  I. production of bile
 II. synthesis of amino acids
III. gluconeogenesis

  (A) I and II
  (B) I and III
  (C) II and III
  (D) I, II, and III

40. Which substance causes contraction of the gallbladder?

(A) secretin
(B) cholecystokinin
(C) bilirubin
(D) bile salts

41. What is one of the main components of bile?

(A) bilirubin
(B) degenerated hepatic cells
(C) cholecystokinin
(D) pancreatic lipase

42. A 39-year-old female complains of right lower quadrant pain. Prior to performing an abdominal assessment, in what order should you consider performing the following assessment techniques?

(A) inspection, palpation, and auscultation
(B) palpation, auscultation, and inspection
(C) inspection, auscultation, and palpation
(D) auscultation, palpation, and inspection

43. Depression of overall protein stores is commonly monitored during a nutritional assessment. Which of the following are measured as part of the routine protein assessment during an analysis of nutritional status?

  I. total lymphocytes
  II. albumin
  III. lactate

    (A) I and II
    (B) I and III
    (C) II and III
    (D) I, II, and III

44. A 76-year-old male is receiving tube feeding supplements consisting of Osmolite at 75 cc/h. Approximately how many calories are being administered every 24 hours based on this feeding rate?

(A) 1200 kcal
(B) 1800 kcal
(C) 2400 kcal
(D) 3000 kcal

45. Vomiting of blood from the gastrointestinal system is denoted by which of the following terms?

(A) hemoptysis
(B) hematemesis
(C) hematopol
(D) hematochezia

46. At which anatomic location do most ulcers occur?

(A) stomach
(B) duodenem
(C) esophagus
(D) jejunum

47. Which of the following is thought to be the most common cause of stress ulcers?

(A) ischemia
(B) excessive acid production
(C) mechanical injury
(D) infections

48. Hydrogen ion blocking agents, such as cimetidine (Tagamet) and ranitidine (Zantac), work by which of the following mechanisms?

(A) decreasing gastric acid production
(B) supplying a protective membrane against hydrochloric acid
(C) increasing bicarbonate production
(D) blocking the release of catabolic hydrogen enzymes

49. Which of the following treatments is NOT routinely indicated in the treatment of upper gastrointestinal bleeding?

(A) endoscopy with coagulation of bleeding site
(B) fluid replacement with crystalloids
(C) blood transfusions
(D) iced lavage of the stomach

50. Esophageal varices are the result of increases in which of the following vascular parameters?

(A) hepatic arterial pressure
(B) hepatic venous pressure
(C) portal venous pressure
(D) superior iliac arterial pressure

51. Portacaval shunts work to decrease bleeding from esophageal varices by which mechanism?

(A) decreasing portal venous pressure
(B) improving vena caval blood flow
(C) improving production of clotting factors
(D) decreasing blood return to the liver

Questions 52 and 53 refer to the following scenario.

A 61-year-old male is admitted to your unit with the diagnosis of upper gastrointestinal bleeding. He has a history of alcohol abuse and prior gastrointestinal bleeding. His abdomen is distended and his liver is enlarged. He has no complaints of pain. The vomitus is bright red in color.

52. Based on the preceding information, which condition is most likely to be present?

(A) diverticuli
(B) esophageal varices
(C) duodenal ulcers
(D) colonic varices

53. The physician elects to place an esophageal balloon (Sengstaken-Blakemore) to aid bleeding control. Which of the following is NOT a potential complication of the esophageal balloon treatment?

(A) tracheal occlusion
(B) esophageal necrosis
(C) esophageal rupture
(D) reversal of portal blood flow

54. Which of the following is NOT a commmon cause of lower gastrointestinal bleeding?

(A) diverticulosis
(B) colon tumors
(C) arteriovenous malformations
(D) hepatic failure

55. Which of the following is NOT a treatment for lower gastrointestinal tract bleeding?

(A) vasopressin
(B) endoscopy
(C) colon resection
(D) balloon tamponade

56. A 57-year-old male with the diagnosis of hepatitis A is admitted to your unit. He is also recovering from vascular surgery and has an open wound on his left lower leg. Which type of isolation is likely to be requested for this patient?

(A) enteric
(B) respiratory
(C) wound
(D) reverse

57. A 69-year-old male has been in your unit for 31 days following an episode of acute respiratory failure. He is receiving nutritional supplementation consisting of 50 cc/hr of Pulmocare. His current laboratory information is as follows:

albumin	2.4 g/dL
white blood cell count	4500 mm^3
lymphocytes	20%
Na$^+$	130 mEq/L

Based on the preceding information, what is the total lymphocyte count?

(A) 200 mm^3
(B) 900 mm^3
(C) 2000 mm^3
(D) 2800 mm^3

Questions 58 and 59 refer to the following scenario.

A 23-year-old female is admitted to your unit after being found unresponsive by paramedics. She has no overt signs of injury or physical abuse. After starting an intravenous drip, you accidentally stick yourself with the same needle used for the venipuncture.

58. Based on the preceding information, to what type of hepatitis would you most likely be exposed?

(A) hepatitis A
(B) hepatitis B
(C) non-A, non-B hepatitis
(D) hepatitis D

59. Initial treatment for you, assuming no prior exposure to hepatitis exists, would include administration of which of the following (after appropriate serologic studies of you and the patient had been performed)?

    (A) hepatitis B immune globulin (HBIG) and vaccine
    (B) hepatitis A immune globulin (HAIG)
    (C) non-A, non-B hepatitis immune globulin
    (D) hepatitis A vaccine

60. For which type of hepatitis does an effective vaccine exist?

    (A) hepatitis A
    (B) hepatitis B
    (C) non-A, non-B hepatitis
    (D) hepatitis D

Questions 61 and 62 refer to the following scenario.

A 67-year-old male is admitted to your unit with the complaints of generalized fatigue and weakness. His abdomen is distended with ascites present, producing shortness of breath. The liver is hard but not enlarged. Spider angiomas are noted on his chest and he has atrophied skeletal muscles. Sclera have an icteric appearance. Vital signs are blood pressure 96/60, pulse 110, and respiratory rate 28.

61. Based on the preceding information, which condition is likely to be responsible for the symptoms?

    (A) acute hepatitis
    (B) cirrhosis
    (C) esophageal varices
    (D) hepatorenal syndrome

62. Which initial treatment would be indicated to help relieve the respiratory distress from the ascites?

    (A) placing the patient in a supine position
    (B) endoscopy
    (C) protein restriction in the diet
    (D) administration of diuretics and sodium restriction

63. All of the following are nursing measures for the patient with acute hepatitis except one. Which one is NOT indicated in the patient with hepatitis?

    (A) low-protein, high-carbohydrate diet
    (B) monitoring liver enzyme tests
    (C) maximizing periods of rest
    (D) avoiding periods of rest, initiating active exercise regimes

64. Asterixis is regarded as a sign of the development of which condition?

(A) left ventricular failure
(B) acute calcium disturbance
(C) hepatic encephalopathy
(D) seizures

Questions 65 and 66 refer to the following scenario.

A 53-year-old male is admitted to the unit with the diagnosis of cirrhosis. He currently is confused and disoriented. He has a "flapping" movement of both hands and has jaundiced skin. Laboratory values are as follows:

SGOT	100
SGPT	88
LDH	250
alkaline phosphatase	165

65. Based on the preceding information, which condition is likely to be developing and causing the behavioral changes?

(A) acute renal failure
(B) loss of cerebral perfusion pressure
(C) loss of cerebral glucose from hepatic failure
(D) hepatic encephalopathy

66. Which treatment would be utilized in the treatment of this patient?

(A) lactulose
(B) high-protein diet
(C) glucose bolus
(D) vitamin D and B administration

67. Pancreatitis is partially monitored by means of which parameters?

(A) pepsinogen levels
(B) amylase values
(C) glucagon values
(D) trypsin levels

68. What is the most common cause of pancreatitis?

(A) liver failure
(B) diabetes
(C) alcohol abuse
(D) intravenous drug abuse

Questions 69 and 70 refer to the following scenario.

A 46-year-old male, with a history of alcohol abuse, is admitted to your unit with the development of severe abdominal pain, with radiation of the pain to his back. The abdomen is tender although rebound tenderness in not present. He is nauseated and has vomited once. Bowel sounds are diminished. Vital signs are blood pressure 98/58, pulse 116, and respiratory rate 34. Laboratory data are as follows:

Na^+	142
K^+	3.8
Cl^-	106
HCO_3^-	22
Ca^{2+}	7.5
Amylase	600

69. Based on the preceding information, which condition is likely to be developing?

    (A) superior mesenteric obstruction
    (B) cholecystitis
    (C) pancreatitis
    (D) bowel obstruction

70. Which treatment, aside from pain relief, would be indicated for this patient?

    (A) placement on an NPO (*non per os*; nothing by mouth) regime with gastrointestinal suction
    (B) reduction in the quantity of nitrogen-containing products in the diet
    (C) exploratory laparotomy
    (D) cholecystectomy

71. Which of the following electrolytes is frequently lost with pancreatitis?

    (A) sodium
    (B) potassium
    (C) bicarbonate
    (D) calcium

Questions 72 and 73 refer to the following scenario.

A 69-year-old female is admitted to your unit complaining of excruciating periumbilical pain. Her abdomen is not tender although she does exhibit rebound tenderness. All laboratory values are normal. Vital signs are blood pressure 168/92, pulse 113, and respiratory rate 28.

72. Based on the preceding information, which condition is most likely to be developing?

(A) superior mesenteric arterial obstruction
(B) cholecystitis
(C) pancreatitis
(D) bowel obstruction

73. Which treatment, aside from pain relief, would be indicated for this patient?

(A) placement on an NPO (*non per os*; nothing by mouth) regime with gastrointestinal suction
(B) endoscopy with cauterization
(C) laparotomy with possible mesenteric embolectomy
(D) cholecystectomy

Questions 74 and 75 refer to the following scenario.

A 76-year-old female is admitted to your unit with vomiting, nausea, and diffuse abdominal pain. The vomitus has a fecal odor. She had a cholecystectomy in the past but has been in good health until the development of abdominal pain two days ago. The abdomen has a hyperresonant sound on percussion, with the patient complaining of tenderness to palpation. Laboratory data are normal.

74. Based on the preceding information, which condition is likely to be developing?

(A) bowel obstruction
(B) mesenteric artery occlusion
(C) pyloric stenosis
(D) obstruction of the pancreatic duct

75. Treatment for this condition most likely would include which of the following?

(A) endoscopy for pyloric valve repair
(B) endoscopy with embolectomy of the pancreatic head
(C) laparotomy with possible mesenteric embolectomy
(D) laparotomy for relief of obstruction

76. All of the following can cause intestinal perforation. Which is the most common cause of intestinal perforation?

(A) bowel obstruction
(B) appendicitis
(C) colonic ulcers
(D) gastric ulcers

Questions 77 and 78 refer to the following scenario.

A 29-year-old male is admitted to your unit with complaints of generalized abdominal pain. The pain started yesterday and became worse, but then improved, before worsening again this morning. An abdominal examination reveals diffuse tenderness and "boardlike" rigidity with the patient preferring not to move. An abdominal x-ray reveals free air under the diaphragm. Laboratory data reveal the following:

Na^+	141
K^+	4.2
Cl^-	99
HCO_3^-	25
Amylase	50
WBC	13,000

77. Based on the preceding information, which condition is likely to be present?

    (A) pancreatitis
    (B) superior mesenteric artery obstruction
    (C) intestinal perforation
    (D) cholecystitis

78. Which treatment would be indicated for this condition?

    (A) placement on an NPO (*non per os*; nothing by mouth) regime with gastrointestinal suction
    (B) sedation with narcotics while waiting for the pain to subside
    (C) upper and lower endoscopy to search for obstructions
    (D) exploratory laparotomy

CHAPTER 5

Renal Practice Exam

1. A 24-year-old female is admitted to your unit following a fall from a 3-foot ladder. She landed on her posterior right side and complains of pain between T-7 and T-12. She is alert and oriented and has no difficulty breathing. Based on the preceding information, which organ is most likely to have been injured?

   (A) spleen
   (B) kidney
   (C) pancreas
   (D) descending colon

2. Which of the following is/are NOT located in the renal cortex?

   (A) glomeruli
   (B) distal convoluted tubules
   (C) proximal convoluted tubules
   (D) loop of Henle

3. Which arteriole is the primary arterial branch entering the glomerulus?

   (A) afferent
   (B) efferent
   (C) cortex
   (D) vasa recta

4. Which part of the nephron immediately leaves the glomerulus?

   (A) distal convoluted tubule
   (B) proximal convoluted tubule
   (C) afferent arteriole
   (D) juxtaglomerular apparatus

5. The right kidney is slightly lower than the left. What is the reason for this difference?

(A) the right kidney is larger due to the presence of more nephronal structures
(B) the left kidney is displaced upward by the spleen
(C) the right kidney is displaced downward by the liver
(D) the left kidney is drawn upward by the diaphragm

6. The kidneys have the ability to regulate blood flow partially via local regulatory mechanisms. If the systemic blood pressure falls, how does the kidney maintain perfusion?

(A) decreasing nephronal resistance to glomerular filtrate
(B) afferent arteriole dilation and efferent arteriole constriction
(C) efferent arteriole dilation and afferent arteriole constriction
(D) decreasing glomerular filtration rate and increase active secretion levels

7. Fluid is forced from the glomerulus, forming an ultrafiltrate. Into which compartment is the fluid forced?

(A) Bowman's capsule
(B) proximal tubule
(C) collecting ducts
(D) distal tubule

8. Which of the following elements is NOT filtered during glomerular filtration?

(A) sodium
(B) potassium
(C) proteins
(D) creatinine

9. From a renal perspective, secretion can be defined by which of the following descriptions?

(A) movement of solutes and water from the peritubular network into the tubule
(B) movement of solutes and water from the tubule into the peritubular network
(C) movement of high-molecular-weight particles into the urine
(D) acceleration of electrolyte elimination at the glomerulus

10. Glomerular filtration is affected by all of the following factors. Which has the most significant effect on glomerular filtration rate?

(A) osmotic pressure of the blood
(B) hydrostatic pressure of the blood
(C) dilation of the afferent arteriole
(D) constriction of the efferent arteriole

Questions 11 and 12 refer to the following scenario.

A 37-year-old male is in your unit following a motor vehicle accident. During the initial 24 hours, he was hypotensive and developed acute renal failure. His current laboratory data reveal the following information:

urinary osmolality	510 mosm
urinary Na+	51 mEq/L
serum osmolality	298 mEq/L
serum Na+	126 mEq/L

11. Based on the preceding information, which condition is likely to be present?

(A) dehydration
(B) fluid overload
(C) acute renal failure
(D) glomerulonephritis

12. Which laboratory data are abnormal?

   I. serum Na+
  II. urinary osmolality
 III. serum osmolality
  IV. urinary Na+

   (A) I
   (B) I and III
   (C) II and IV
   (D) IV

13. Which of the following corresponds most closely to normal serum osmolality?

(A) 50 to 100 mosm
(B) 100 to 250 mosm
(C) 280 to 320 mosm
(D) 320 to 410 mosm

14. Which of the following corresponds most closely to the range of normal serum sodium values?

(A) 40 to 60 mEq/L
(B) 60 to 75 mEq/L
(C) 80 to 120 mEq/L
(D) 135 to 145 mEq/L

15. Which of the following corresponds most closely to the range of normal serum potassium values?

(A) 1 to 2 mEq/L
(B) 2.5 to 3.5 mEq/L
(C) 3.5 to 5.0
(D) 5 to 6.5 mEq/L

16. Which of the following corresponds most closely to the range of normal urine sodium values?

(A) 40 to 220 mEq/L
(B) 220 to 320 mEq/L
(C) 335 to 445 mEq/L
(D) 455 to 470 mEq/L

17. Which of the following corresponds most closely to the range of normal serum calcium levels?

(A) 1 to 3 mg/dL
(B) 4.5 to 6.5 mg/dL
(C) 6 to 8 mg/dL
(D) 8.5 to 10.5 mg/dL

18. An 81-year-old male has been in the intensive care unit for 45 days secondary to surgical complications from a ruptured bowel. The physician suspects that he may have nutritional impairment despite hyperalimentation. Laboratory tests reveal the following serum electrolyte information:

Na^+	141 mEq/L
K^+	3.9 mEq/L
Cl^-	102 mEq/L
HCO_3^-	25 mEq/L
Ca^{2+}	8.9 mg/dL
Mg^{2+}	4.3 mg/dL

Which of the preceding laboratory valves is/are abnormal?

(A) Mg^{2+}
(B) Ca^{2+}
(C) Cl^- and Na^+
(D) K^+ and HCO_3^-

19. Which of the following corresponds most closely to the range of normal phosphate levels?

    (A) 3 to 4.5 mg/dL
    (B) 4.5 to 6.5 mg/dL
    (C) 6 to 8 mg/dL
    (D) 8.5 to 10.5 mg/dL

20. Creatinine level is a valuable indicator of glomerular filtration rate for which reason?

    (A) Once filtered in the glomerulus, creatinine is not reabsorbed in the tubular system.
    (B) Creatinine only enters the glomerulus when glomerular filtration pressures exceed 60 mm Hg.
    (C) Creatinine filtration is unaffected by renal disease.
    (D) Creatinine is formed in the glomerulus and only decreases in filtration causing creatinine levels to change.

21. What is the effect of ADH (antidiuretic hormone) on renal function?

    (A) It inhibits water reabsorption in the distal tubules and collecting ducts.
    (B) It increases water reabsorption in the distal tubles and collecting ducts.
    (C) It increases fluid excretion from the glomerulus.
    (D) It blocks the effect of loop diuretics, such as Lasix.

22. Which of the following would stimulate the release of ADH (antidiuretic hormone)?

    (A) decreased serum osmolality
    (B) increased serum osmolality
    (C) increased serum creatinine
    (D) decreased urine sodium

23. The countercurrent mechanism in the nephron is designed to accomplish which purpose?

    (A) retaining creatinine
    (B) eliminating hydrogen ions
    (C) concentrating urine
    (D) increasing water loss

24. Most water reabsorption occurs in which part of the nephron?

(A) proximal tubules
(B) loop of Henle
(C) distal tubules
(D) collecting ducts

25. A 46-year-old male is in your unit following an episode of ARD (acute respiratory distress) after radiation therapy for large cell lung cancer. His urine output decreases on day 3 of his intensive care unit stay to 20 cc/hour. The physician asks you to call him if the patient's BUN (blood urea nitrogen)/creatinine ratio becomes abnormal. The following laboratory data are available:

serum BUN	64
serum creatinine	2
urine Na+	76

Based on this information, is the BUN/creatinine ratio abnormal and should you contact the physician?

(A) The BUN/creatinine level is normal; do not call the physician.
(B) The BUN/creatinine level is low; call the physician.
(C) The BUN/creatinine level is high; call the physician.
(D) BUN/creatinine ratios cannot be calculated without urinary creatinine and BUN values.

26. Which of the following corresponds most closely to the range of normal serum creatinine levels?

(A) 0.8 to 1.8
(B) 2 to 2.9
(C) 3.2 to 4
(D) 4.5 to 5

27. Which of the following corresponds most closely to the range of normal serum BUN levels?

(A) 10 to 20 mg/dL
(B) 20 to 30 mg/dL
(C) 30 to 40 mg/dL
(D) 40 to 50 mg/dL

28. In the presence of oliguria, a BUN/creatinine ratio greater than normal suggests that which condition has developed?

(A) prerenal failure
(B) renal failure
(C) postrenal failure
(D) acute tubular necrosis

29. Aldosterone exerts an effect on renal function at which anatomic site?

(A) proximal tubule
(B) loop of Henle
(C) distal tubule
(D) glomerulus

30. The juxtaglomerulur system is responsible for releasing which substance?

(A) erythropoietin
(B) aldosterone
(C) secretin
(D) angiotensin

31. Angiotension II exerts which of the following physiologic actions?

(A) vasoconstriction
(B) vasodilation
(C) increases glomerular filtration rate
(D) promotes ADH (antidiuretic hormone) secretion

32. A 34-year-old male with chronic renal failure has a hemoglobin level of 7.4 g/dL and a hematocrit of 23%. His blood pressure is 160/92 and his heart rate is 98. What is the most likely explanation for the hemoglobin and hemotocrit values?

(A) The values are abnormally elevated due to hemoconcentration.
(B) The values are abnormally low due to a reduced cardiac output.
(C) The values are normal.
(D) The values are decreased due to loss of erythropoietin.

33. Which substance has the most significant effect on sodium regulation?

(A) renin level
(B) aldosterone level
(C) glomerular filtration rate
(D) serum pH

34. What is the primary action of aldosterone?

(A) inhibits sodium excretion
(B) promotes sodium excretion
(C) blocks water reabsorption
(D) stimulates vasoconstriction

35. What is the primary cause of hypernatremia?

(A) vascular water deficits
(B) excessive vascular free water
(C) excessive serum sodium levels
(D) loss of serum chloride

36. The lack of ADH (antidiuretic hormone) causes which effect on serum electrolytes?

(A) increase in sodium levels
(B) decrease in sodium levels
(C) decrease in hydrogen ion levels
(D) increase in serum bicarbonate levels

37. Which of the following is NOT a common sign of hypernatremia?

(A) tachycardia
(B) dry mucous membranes
(C) poor skin turgor
(D) distended neck veins

38. Administration of which of the following is a normal initial treatment for hypernatremia?

(A) diuretics
(B) nonelectrolyte (free water) solutions
(C) normal saline
(D) potassium salts

39. Hyponatremia is most often caused by which of the following?

(A) excessive sodium levels
(B) decreased sodium levels
(C) excessive vascular volume
(D) decreased vascular volume

40. The most dangerous symptoms of hyponatremia center on which organ system?

(A) central nervous system
(B) cardiac system
(C) renal system
(D) respiratory system

41. Excessive secretion of ADH (antidiuretic hormone) could produce which of the following electrolyte changes?

  I. decreased serum osmolality
  II. increased serum sodim
  III. decreased serum sodium

    (A) I
    (B) II
    (C) II and III
    (D) I and III

42. Treatment of severe hyponatremia (<120 mEq/L) consists of administration of which of the following?

    (A) diuretics
    (B) nonelectrolyte (free water) solutions
    (C) normal saline
    (D) potassium salts

43. Hypokalemia is associated with which acid-base disturbance?

    (A) metabolic acidosis
    (B) metabolic alkalosis
    (C) respiratory acidosis
    (D) systemic acidosis

44. Which of the following ECG (electrocardiographic) changes is NOT associated with hyperkalemia?

    (A) peaked T waves
    (B) depressed P waves
    (C) PVCs (premature ventricular contractions)
    (D) widening QRS complex

45. Which of the following is NOT recommended for the treatment of hyperkalemia?

    (A) Kayexalate
    (B) glucose/insulin infusion
    (C) dialysis
    (D) ammonium chloride

46. Hypokalemia is associated with which of the following ECG changes?

(A) peaked T waves
(B) depressed P waves
(C) PVCs (premature ventricular contractions)
(D) widening QRS complex

47. The concentration of which electrolyte is inversely related to that of calcium?

(A) sodium
(B) potassium
(C) phosphate
(D) magnesium

48. Which mechanism is calcium NOT involved in regulating?

(A) coagulation
(B) formation of bone
(C) transmission of electrical impulses
(D) absorption of vitamin D

49. A 51-year-old male with a history of alcoholism has marked muscle irritability. The following laboratory data are available:

Na^+	135 mEq/L
K^+	4.8 mEq/L
Ca^{2+}	3.7 mg/dL
Mg^{2+}	1.8 mg/dL

Which of the following electrolytes is most likely to be the source of the muscle hyperirritability?

(A) sodium
(B) calcium
(C) potassium
(D) magnesium

50. Chvostek's sign is tested by which maneuver?

(A) tapping the flexor tendon over the knee
(B) tapping the supramandibular area
(C) stroking the sole of the foot
(D) measuring clotting times after venipuncture

51. Trousseau's sign is a test for which electrolyte deficiency?

(A) hypophosphatemia
(B) hypercalcemia
(C) hypocalcemia
(D) hypokalemia

52. Which organ or organ system is involved in the regulation of phosphate elimination?

(A) liver
(B) respiratory system
(C) renal system
(D) spleen

53. A 75-year-old female is admitted to your unit with pneumonia and malnutrition. Her chief complaint currently is weakness and inability to perform her normal "chores." She has stated that she has not eaten well for the past several months. The following information is available:

Na^+	150 mEq/L
K^+	3.6 mEq/L
Cl^-	110 mEq/L
Mg^{2+}	2.1 mg/dL
Ca^{2+}	9.2 mg/dL
PO_4^{3-}	2.3 mg/dL

Which of the preceding levels is a likely source of her weakness?

(A) low phosphate
(B) high sodium and chloride
(C) low magnesium
(D) high calcium

54. Which of the following does NOT have phosphate as a component?

(A) ATP (adenosine triphosphate)
(B) ADP (adenosine disphosphate)
(C) 2,3-DPG (2,3-diphosphodiglyceride)
(D) PTH (parathyroid hormone)

55. Which electrolyte is directly related to the reabsorption of magnesium?

(A) potassium
(B) calcium
(C) sodium
(D) phosphate

56. Which of the following is a primary treatment to reduce magnesium levels?

(A) normal saline bolus
(B) dialysis
(C) mechanical ventilation
(D) calcium carbonate administration

57. Hypomagnesemia is manifested clinically by which of the following symptoms?

(A) muscle irritability
(B) muscle fatigue
(C) nausea
(D) positive Turner's sign

58. A 61-year-old male admitted with the diagnosis of COPD (chronic obstructive pulmonary disease) has the following set of laboratory data for arterial blood gases and electrolytes:

PO_2	63 mm Hg
PCO_2	71 mm Hg
pH	7.37
HCO_3^-	39 mEq/L
Na^+	146 mEq/L
Cl^-	87 mEq/L

The COPD-induced blood gas changes have altered the electrolytes as well. Based on the preceding information, which electrolyte change occurred because of the PCO_2 elevation?

I. bicarbonate increased
II. chloride decreased
III. sodium increased

(A) I
(B) III
(C) I and II
(D) II and III

59. Elevated chloride levels are associated with which condition?

(A) alkalosis
(B) acidosis
(C) hyponatremia
(D) hypercalcemia

60. Left ventricular failure will cause which effect on the BUN/creatinine ratio?

(A) It will cause the ratio to rise.
(B) It will cause the ratio to fall.
(C) It will have no effect on the ratio but will elevate creatinine levels.
(D) It will reverse the ratio.

61. A 74-year-old female is admitted to your unit with possible sepsis and renal failure. The following laboratory information is available:

urinary Na^+	13
urinary osmolarity	1000
urine output	15 cc/hr

Based on these data, what is likely to be occurring?

(A) prerenal azotemia
(B) acute tubular necrosis
(C) postrenal obstruction
(D) vasomotor nephropathy

62. A 61-year-old female is in your unit after being admitted from a nursing home. At the time of admission, it was noted that she seemed confused, although she is currently alert and oriented. She has had a "cold" for the past several days. Her laboratory data are as follows:

Na^+	155
K^+	3.6
Cl^-	122
HCO_3^-	24

What is the most likely reason for the abnormal sodium level?

(A) excess total sodium
(B) decreased total potassium
(C) dehydration
(D) fluid excess

63. Which of the following patients has an increased anion gap?

	1	2	3	4
Na^+	132	142	121	153
K^+	3.2	4.8	4.1	3.5
Cl^-	93	108	89	113
HCO_3^-	25	17	19	26

(A) patient 1
(B) patient 2
(C) patient 3
(D) patient 4

64. What is the clinical value in establishing whether or not an anion gap exists?

(A) The finding permits determination of a metabolic alkalosis.
(B) The finding permits determination of a metabolic acidosis.
(C) The finding permits identification of respiratory acidosis.
(D) The anion gap acts as a marker of acute renal failure.

Questions 65 and 66 refer to the following scenario.

A 61-year-old male has a two-day history of abdominal pain with nausea and vomiting. He has intermittent chest pain, which is unrelieved by nitrates, changes in position, or rest. He has a history of CHF (congestive heart failure) and underwent a CABG (coronary artery bypass graft) two years ago. Currently he has a urine output of 15 cc/hr. He has had a urine output of 200 cc over the past 24 hours. Currently he has the following vital signs:

blood pressure	88/56
pulse	114
respiratory rate	32

He has a pulmonary artery catheter in place, from which the following information is available:

CO	3.7
CI	2.4
PA	20/8
PCWP	6
CVP	2

The following laboratory data are also available:

SMA-6	
Na^+	153
K^+	3.6
Cl^-	120
HCO_3^-	19
creatinine	2.2
glucose	154
BUN	35
osmolality	320

He has the following blood gas values:

PaO_2	82
$PaCO_2$	28
pH	7.30

HCO_3^-	20
SvO_2	52%
PvO_2	32

Urinary electrolyte values are as follows:

Na^+	35
osmolality	845
creatinine	48

Other laboratory data include the following:

albumin	3.6
hemoglobin	15.6
lactate	2.2

65. Based on the preceding information, what is the potential problem and the likely reason for the decrease in urine output?

   (A) prerenal azotemia from hypovolemia
   (B) prerenal azotemia from left ventricular failure
   (C) acute tubular necrosis
   (D) ATN from hypovolemia

66. What would be the most effective therapy to improve this patient's renal function?

   (A) fluid bolus
   (B) dobutamine therapy
   (C) diuretics
   (D) renal dose dopamine

67. A 31-year-old female is in the intensive care unit following multiple gunshot wounds to her face and abdomen. She has been in the unit for four days and during the fourth day her urine output decreases to 200 cc for the entire day. She is alert and oriented yet cannot communicate because of an endotracheal tube. The following information is available to you:

Na^+	132
K^+	4.1
Cl^-	99
HCO_3^-	20
creatinine	2.5
BUN	43
osmolality	295
urinary creatinine	50
urinary osmolality	343

Based on the preceding information, what is the most likely cause of her decreased urine output?

    (A) prerenal azotemia from hypovolemia
    (B) prerenal azotemia from rhabdomyolysis
    (C) acute tubular necrosis
    (D) ureter obstruction

68. As you are orienting a preceptor, she asks you about the treatment your patient is receiving for an infection. She tells you she remembers being taught that aminoglycosides (your patient is receiving gentamycin) can cause renal failure. Yet your patient has a normal urine output (2100 cc/day) and the following laboratory values:

Na^+	142
K^+	4.6
Cl^-	103
HCO_3^-	21
creatinine	3.2
BUN	54
osmolality	278
urinary osmolality	297
urinary Na^+	49

She asks if this patient is at any risk for developing renal failure. Based on the preceding information, what would you answer?

    (A) As long as the urine output is greater than 30 mL/hr she is not in danger of renal failure.
    (B) As long as her creatinine level is no greater than 2.5 mg/dL she is not at risk for acute renal failure.
    (C) Based on the information, she already has signs of acute renal failure.
    (D) Although she may be at risk for renal failure, a renal ultrasound scan would be required to make a definitive diagnosis.

69. A 65-year-old male is in the intensive care unit for a CVA (cerebrovascular accident) and possible CHF (congestive heart failure) secondary to systemic hypertension. He is currently intubated after developing a respiratory acidosis in the emergency room. During the second day in the unit, he begins to put out over 2000 cc of urine on your shift. The following laboratory information is available:

Na^+	158
K^+	3.4
Cl^-	112

HCO_3^-	23
creatinine	1.8
BUN	29
osmolality	341
urinary osmolality	343
urinary Na^+	28

Based on the preceding information, what condition is likely to be developing?

(A) prerenal azotemia
(B) acute renal failure
(C) diabetes insipidus
(D) inappropriate secretion of ADH (antidiuretic hormone)

70. Measurement of which of the following is helpful in differentiating acute renal failure from PRA (prerenal azotemia)?

I. FENa
II. BUN
III. urinary osmolality

(A) I and II
(B) I and III
(C) II and III
(D) I, II, and III

71. During the care of a patient undergoing peritoneal dialysis, the infusate has not completely drained. Which method would be acceptable to help facilitate drainage?

(A) applying continuous low-pressure suction
(B) turning the patient from side to side
(C) manipulating the peritoneal catheter
(D) applying manual pressure to the abdomen

72. Which of the following is NOT considered an indication for continuous arteriovenous hemofiltration?

(A) treating acute volume overload in congestive heart failure
(B) fluid removal when diuretic therapy has failed
(C) acute hyperkalemia
(D) as a replacement for hemodialysis in the non–university hospital setting

73. Which of the following will continuous arteriovenous hemofiltration NOT remove?

   (A) fluid
   (B) albumin
   (C) sodium
   (D) potassium

Questions 74 and 75 refer to the following scenario.

A 72-year-old male is in your unit with chronic CHF (congestive heart failure). He has become increasingly resistant to diuretic therapy. CAVH (continuous arteriovenous hemofiltration) is started to help alleviate his symptoms. After one day on CAVH, the filtrate from the CAVH begins to diminish. The arteriovenous filter is warm to the touch and pulsates with each pulse. You notice that the filter is on an IV pole about 12 inches above the patient's heart level. His blood pressure is 100/62, pulse 98, respiratory rate 24, temperature 37.5° C.

74. Based on the preceding information, which condition is likely to be developing?

   (A) inadequacy of pump inflow rates
   (B) obstruction of the CAVH filter
   (C) obstruction of the arteriovenous catheter
   (D) inadequate arterial pressure

75. What measures could you take to correct the situation?

   (A) add potassium to the dialysate until the flow problem is corrected
   (B) add glucose to the dialysate to develop an osmotic pressure gradient
   (C) increase the outflow pump rate
   (D) lower the filter to heart level

CHAPTER 6 _____

Endocrine Practice Exam

1. An increase in hormone concentration will cause which of the following?

   (A) an inhibition of hormone releasing factors
   (B) an increase of hormone releasing factors
   (C) increased production by the pituitary
   (D) increased production by the hypothalamus

2. The hormones of the adrenal medulla are under the control of which structure?

   (A) hypothalamus
   (B) posterior pituitary
   (C) anterior pituitary
   (D) autonomic nervous system

3. All of the adenohyphophyseal hormones have an effect on a target gland EXCEPT:

   (A) adrenocorticotropin
   (B) growth hormone
   (C) thyroid-stimulating hormone
   (D) luteinizing hormone

4. The anterior pituitary receives stimulation from the hypothalamus through which of the following?

   (A) vascular system
   (B) sympathetic nervous system
   (C) parasympathetic nervous system
   (D) central nervous system

5. Which of the following is NOT secreted by the anterior pituitary gland:

   (A) ACTH (adrenocorticotropic hormone)
   (B) thyroid-stimulating hormone
   (C) growth hormone
   (D) ADH (antidiuretic hormone)

6. Which of the following is a factor inhibiting the release of growth hormone?

   (A) hypoglycemia
   (B) exercise
   (C) hyperglycemia
   (D) decreased amino acid levels

7. ADH (antidiuretic hormone) release is inhibited by which of the following?

   (A) increased serum osmolality
   (B) decreased serum osmolality
   (C) increased serum sodium
   (D) increased potassium level

Questions 8 and 9 refer to the following scenario.

A 25-year-old male is admitted to the intensive care unit with a diagnosis of brainstem contusion. Two days after admission, the patient is consistently thirsty. You note that the urine output is nearly 2000 cc in eight hours with an intake of 950 cc. Blood pressure is 140/74, pulse 84, and respiratory rate 22. The following laboratory data are available:

SERUM		URINE	
Na^+	155	Na^+	14
K^+	3.7	Osmolality	312
Cl^-	114	Specific gravity	1.008
HCO_3^-	23		

8. Based on the preceding information, which condition is likely to be developing?

   (A) SIADH (syndrome of inappropriate antidiuretic hormone secretion)
   (B) adult-onset diabetes mellitus
   (C) anterior pituitary stimulation
   (D) diabetes insipidus

9. Which treatment could be expected to be given to this patient?

(A) Desmopresin acetate (DDAVP, 1-desamino-8-D-arginine vasopressin)
(B) D_5W in a 200-cc/hour fluid bolus
(C) diuretics
(D) fluid restriction

10. A patient is admitted to the intensive care unit with a diagnosis of SIADH (syndrome of inappropriate antidiuretic hormone secretion). Which laboratory data would be expected if this diagnosis is correct?

    (A) hyponatremia
    (B) hypernatremia
    (C) increased serum osmolality
    (D) hyperkalemia

11. A common clinical finding of SIADH (syndrome of inappropriate antidiuretic hormone secretion) may include which symptom?

    (A) mental status changes
    (B) tachycardia
    (C) polyuria
    (D) polydipsia

12. Which of the following treatment modalities would NOT be an appropriate treatment modality for SIADH (syndrome of inappropriate antidiuretic hormone secretion)?

    (A) fluid restriction
    (B) diuretic administration
    (C) administration of normal saline
    (D) Kayexalate enemas

13. The critical care nurse should recognize that a major complication of diabetes insipidus could include:

    (A) dehydration
    (B) hyponatremia
    (C) hyperkalemia
    (D) bradycardia and hypertension

14. What is the dominant effect of ADH (antidiuretic hormone) on the kidneys?

    (A) It causes them to excrete water and sodium.
    (B) It causes them to reabsorb water and concentrate urine.
    (C) It causes them to reabsorb sodium and excrete potassium.
    (D) It causes them to reabsorb potassium and excrete sodium.

15. Which hormone(s) does the thyroid gland NOT secrete?

(A) thyroxine
(B) triiodothyronine
(C) calcitonin
(D) ADH (antidiuretic hormone)

16. The release of thyroxine is inhibited by which situation?

(A) hyperthermia
(B) hyperglycemia
(C) hypokalemia
(D) hypernatremia

17. Calcitonin is released by which organ?

(A) pituitary gland
(B) adrenal gland
(C) parathyroid gland
(D) thyroid gland

18. Which of the following is another name for hyperthyroidism?

(A) myxedema coma
(B) Graves's disease
(C) hirsuitism
(D) Lugol's syndrome

Questions 19 and 20 refer to the following scenario.

A 48-year-old female is admitted to your unit with a possible syncopal episode. She is currently awake although she is nervous and anxious. Vital signs are as follows:

blood pressure	178/108
pulse	129
respiratory rate	28
temperature	39° C

During your initial examination, you note that she has exophthalmos and that her skin is warm and wet.

19. Given the preceding information, which condition could be present?

(A) myxedema coma
(B) parathyroid crisis
(C) thyroid storm
(D) aldosterone crisis

20. Which of the following would be administered in this situation?

(A) calcitonin
(B) propranolol (Inderal)
(C) normal saline
(D) parathyroid hormone

21. On which organ does calcitonin exert its major effect?

(A) kidney
(B) bone
(C) parathyroid
(D) liver

22. Parathormone release is inhibited by which serum situation?

(A) increased calcium
(B) decreased magnesium
(C) increased phosphate
(D) increased magnesium

23. Parathormone secretion is stimulated by which humoral event?

(A) decreased calcium
(B) increased magnesium
(C) increased phosphate
(D) all of the above

24. Which of the following is a symptom of hypothyroidism?

(A) paresthesia of the fingers
(B) sensitivity to cold
(C) dry, scaly skin
(D) all of the above

25. Which of the following is NOT a symptom of myxedema coma?

(A) hypothermia
(B) hypoventilation
(C) hyponatremia
(D) hyperthermia

Questions 26 and 27 refer to the following scenario.

A 51-year-old female is admitted to your unit with hypotension, bradycardia, and decreased level of consciousness. Her core temperature is 35.5°C. The temperature in her apartment was 25°C (77°F). No history is available regarding prior medical problems. She appears to be overweight, with dry, scaly skin and puffy face and lips. Blood gases analysis reveals the following information:

pH	7.25
$PaCO_2$	56
PaO_2	63

Shortly after admission, she has a grand mal seizure. She is intubated and placed on mechanical ventilation.

26. Based on the preceding information, which condition is likely to be developing?

    (A) acute CHF (congestive heart failure)
    (B) ARDS (adult respiratory distress syndrome)
    (C) thyroid crisis
    (D) myxedema coma

27. Which treatment would be required to correct the condition?

    (A) dobutamine (50 mg/kg per min)
    (B) hyperventilation
    (C) levothyroxine (0.3 mg)
    (D) calcitonin (2 mg/kg per h)

28. Which of the following is NOT a common precipitating factor of myxedema coma?

    (A) stress
    (B) exposure to heat
    (C) infection
    (D) exposure to cold

29. Which of the following is NOT a common symptom of hyperthyroidism?

    (A) marked fatigue
    (B) cold intolerance
    (C) tachycardia
    (D) weight loss

30. Which of the following is NOT associated as a precipitating factor with thyrotoxic crisis?

(A) diabetic ketoacidosis
(B) trauma
(C) increased intracranial pressure
(D) infection

31. A deficiency of parathormone causes which clinical sign?

    (A) hypocalcemia
    (B) hypercalcemia
    (C) hyponatremia
    (D) hyperkalemia

32. Appropriate response to treatment of myxedema coma would be illustrated by which of the following changes in physiological parameters?

    (A) increase in $PaCO_2$
    (B) reduction in heart rate
    (C) increase in body temperature
    (D) decrease in pH

33. Which of the following is NOT associated with hypoparathyroidism?

    (A) Trousseau's sign
    (B) thyroidectomy
    (C) hypocalcemia
    (D) gastric ulcers

34. Which part of the endocrine system secretes aldosterone?

    (A) zona glomerulus of the adrenal cortex
    (B) zona fasciculata of the adrenal cortex
    (C) adrenal medulla
    (D) zona reticularis of the adrenal cortex

35. Which hormone is NOT secreted by the adrenal cortex?

    (A) glucocorticoids
    (B) mineralocorticoids
    (C) androgenic hormones
    (D) adrenergic hormones

36. Primary adrenal insufficiency is characterized by which of the following?

    (A) hyperpigmentation
    (B) hypertension
    (C) bradycardia
    (D) skeletal tremors

Questions 37 and 38 refer to the following scenario.

A 35-year-old male is admitted to your unit with hypotension and probable dehydration. He is confused and it is difficult to obtain a history regarding past medical problems. He has multiple hyperpigmented areas on his body. He complains of nausea, abdominal pain, and marked fatigue. Laboratory data reveal the following:

Na^+	154
K^+	5.9
Cl^-	109
HCO_3^-	20
glucose	46

37. Based on the preceding information, which condition is likely to be developing?

    (A) myxedema coma
    (B) adrenal insufficiency
    (C) hyperparathyroid storm
    (D) Cushing's syndrome

38. What treatment would most likely be initiated to reverse all of the above symptoms?

    (A) parathormone administration
    (B) thyronine administration
    (C) glucocorticoids administration
    (D) pituitary extract administration

39. Which of the following is another term for adrenal insufficiency?

    (A) Graves's disease
    (B) myxedema crisis
    (C) Addison's disease
    (D) Cushing's syndrome

40. Aldosterone exerts its action on the distal convoluted tubule to cause which effect?

    (A) potassium reabsorption
    (B) sodium excretion
    (C) sodium reabsorption
    (D) chloride excretion

41. Aldosterone release is stimulated by all of the following EXCEPT:

(A) decreased potassium level
(B) renin-angiotension cascade
(C) increased potassium level
(D) decreased sodium level

42. Which of the following stimulates insulin secretion?

    (A) thyroid hormone
    (B) growth hormone
    (C) glucocorticoids
    (D) prolactin

43. Which term best describes gluconeogenesis?

    (A) utilization of oxygen stores due to deficits of serum glucose
    (B) breakdown of protein
    (C) formation of glucose from other substances
    (D) breakdown of glucose stores in the liver

Questions 44 and 45 refer to the following scenario.

A 67-year-old male is admitted to your unit with a decreased level of consciousness. He was brought to the hospital by the police after being found in a shopping mall "acting strange." He complains of fatigue but is generally disoriented as to time and place. His respiratory rate is deep and rapid. Vital signs and laboratory data are given below:

blood pressure	96/58
pulse	114
respiratory rate	34
glucose	760
osmolality	307
PaO_2	91
$PaCO_2$	20
pH	7.28
Na^+	156
K^+	5.0
HCO_3^-	14

The blood pressure also decreases when changing from a lying to a sitting position.

44. Based on the preceding information, which condition is likely developing?

    (A) adrenal crisis
    (B) thyroid storm
    (C) HHNK (hyperosmolar, hyperglycemic, nonketotic) coma
    (D) DKA (diabetic ketoacidosis)

45. Which of the following would most likely be administered to this patient?

(A) glucocorticoids
(B) thyroxine
(C) sodium bicarbonate
(D) insulin and normal saline

46. Which blood gas change is usually present in DKA (diabetic ketoacidosis)?

(A) respiratory acidosis alone
(B) metabolic acidosis alone
(C) respiratory alkalosis and metabolic acidosis
(D) respiratory acidosis and metabolic alkalosis

47. Initial insulin therapy for DKA (diabetic ketoacidosis) is usually administered by which route?

(A) intravenous bolus
(B) intravenous bolus followed by a continuous infusion
(C) subcutaneously
(D) intramuscularly

48. Presenting signs and symptoms of DKA (diabetic ketoacidosis) could include which of the following?

(A) shallow, slow respirations
(B) decreased urine output
(C) tachycardia and orthostatic hypotension
(D) peripheral edema and dependent pulmonary crackles

49. Insulin therapy brings about which electrolyte change?

(A) increased serum potassium
(B) decreased serum sodium
(C) increased intracellular potassium
(D) decreased intracellular calcium

50. HHNK (hyperosmolar, hyperglycemic, nonketotic) coma is differentiated from DKA (diabetic ketoacidosis) by which of the following?

(A) hyperglycemia
(B) absence of ketosis
(C) serum osmolality
(D) serum potassium levels

Questions 51 and 52 refer to the following scenario.

A 57-year-old female is admitted to the unit following a seizure at home. She has no history of seizures. The family describes the patient as not feeling well for several days and has not eaten or taken fluids normally during this time. Her vital signs and laboratory data are as follows:

blood pressure	92/54
pulse	108
respiratory rate	31
glucose	989
osmolality	389
PaO_2	79
$PaCO_2$	30
pH	7.29
Na^+	149
K^+	3.0
HCO_3^-	20

51. Based on the preceding information, which condition is likely to be developing?

    (A) adrenal crisis
    (B) thyroid storm
    (C) HHNK (hyperosmolar, hyperglycemic, nonketotic) coma
    (D) DKA (diabetic ketoacidosis)

52. Which treatment would most likely be initially administered to this patient?

    (A) glucocorticoids
    (B) continuous insulin drip and osmotic volume expanders
    (C) sodium bicarbonate
    (D) D_5W, normal saline fluid bolus, and intermittent insulin

53. Hyperfunction of the adrenal medulla is referred to as which of the following?

    (A) pheochromocytoma
    (B) Addison's disease
    (C) Graves's disease
    (D) Cushing's syndrome

54. Dehydration in HHNK (hyperosmolar, hyperglycemic, nonketotic) coma is primarily due to which event?

(A) lack of ADH (antidiuretic hormone)
(B) inability of the kidney to concentrate urine
(C) nausea and vomiting
(D) osmotic diuresis from the high glucose level

55. HHNK (hyperosmolar, hyperglycemic, nonketotic) coma is partially differentiated from DKA (diabetic ketoacidosis) by which laboratory test?

(A) hyperglycemia
(B) absence of acidosis
(C) hyperkalemia
(D) serum osmolality

Questions 56 and 57 refer to the following scenario.

A 69-year-old, overweight male is in your unit following resection of a perforated bowel. He has a history of adult onset diabetes and mild hypertension. The patient is alert and oriented with stable vital signs at the beginning of your shift. During your shift he becomes disoriented. His skin is cool and clammy, he has muscle tremors, and he complains of nausea. Serum electrolytes are drawn and the laboratory results are listed below:

Na^+	133
K^+	3.7
Cl^-	100
HCO_3^-	25
glucose	43
osmolality	282

56. Based on the preceding information, which condition is likely to be developing?

(A) hyperosmolar, hyperglycemic, nonketotic acidosis
(B) hypoglycemia
(C) diabetic ketoacidosis
(D) diabetes insipidus

57. Which treatment would most likely be given to this patient?

(A) insulin bolus followed by infusion
(B) glucose (dextrose) bolus (D_{50})
(C) normal saline bolus with potassium
(D) glucocorticoids

58. The clinical situation of large fluctuations in blood glucose, such as hypo-glycemia symptoms in a patient with hyperglycemia, is described by which term?

(A) Somogyi effect
(B) Addison's response
(C) Adams's syndrome
(D) pancreatic flash

59. Which of the following physical signs is more indicative of hypoglycemia rather than hyperglycemia?

(A) cool skin
(B) rapid breathing
(C) warm skin
(D) tachycardia

60. At which blood glucose level does change in mentation begin?

(A) 10 to 20 mg/dL
(B) 20 to 30 mg/dL
(C) 30 to 40 mg/dL
(D) any level below 60 mg/dL

61. High serum glucose levels can directly cause which physical symptom?

(A) increased urine output
(B) decreased urine output
(C) hypotension
(D) decreased respiratory rate

62. Which of the following are symptoms of a pheochromocytoma?

I. hypertension
II. tachycardia
III. hyperglycemia

(A) I and II
(B) II and III
(C) I and III
(D) I, II, and III

CHAPTER 7

Immunology and Hematology Practice Exam

1. Which cell, known as the "helper cell," is vital in activating the immune response?

   (A) segmented neutrophil
   (B) band neutrophil
   (C) T4 lymphocyte
   (D) T8 lymphocyte

2. Which of the following components of the immune system is referred to as "cell-mediated" in its immune response?

   (A) segmented neutrophils
   (B) band neutrophils
   (C) T lymphocytes
   (D) B lymphocytes

3. Which cell plays an active role in suppressing the immune response once the antigenic stimulus has been eliminated?

   (A) segmented neutrophil
   (B) band neutrophil
   (C) T4 lymphocyte
   (D) T8 lymphocyte

4. Which of the following components of the white blood count makes up the largest percent of the differential?

   (A) segmented neutrophils
   (B) band neutrophils
   (C) monocytes
   (D) lymphocytes

5. Which term is used to describe a substance regarded as foreign in terms of the immune response?

(A) antibody
(B) antigen
(C) complement
(D) cytotoxic

6. Which of the following are NOT considered macrophages?

(A) segmented neutrophils
(B) band neutrophils
(C) monocytes
(D) lymphocytes

7. A 71-year-old male is admitted to your unit with recurrent pneumonia. Since the pneumonia was present before, which of the following cells would have the ability to remember the *Hemophilus* antigen from a prior infection?

(A) segmented neutrophils
(B) band neutrophils
(C) lymphocytes
(D) eosinophils

8. A 23-year-old female is in your unit following a motor vehicle accident. During the admission, she develops a urinary tract infection. If this were her first exposure to the bacteria causing the infection, which component of the white blood cell count would be the first to respond to the antigen?

(A) segmented neutrophils
(B) eosinophils
(C) T4 lymphocytes
(D) T8 lymphocytes

9. Which of the following types of cells produce antibodies?

(A) segmented neutrophils
(B) monocytes
(C) B lymphocytes through plasma cells
(D) reticuloendothelial cells

10. Which of the following components of the immune system is referred to as "humorally mediated" in its immune response?

(A) segmented neutrophils
(B) band neutrophils
(C) T lymphocytes
(D) B lymphocytes

Questions 11 and 12 refer to the following scenario.

A 21-year-old male is in your unit for respiratory distress due to reaction to chemotherapy for Hodgkin's disease. The following laboratory information is available:

white blood cells	1,300 mm³
segmented neutrophils	25%
banded neutrophils	10%
lymphocytes	25%
platelets	15,000
activated partial thromboplastin time	100 seconds

11. Based on the preceding information, which complications should you be aware may may occur in this situation?

    I. bleeding
    II. infection
    III. hypercoagulation
    (A) I
    (B) I and II
    (C) III
    (D) II and III

12. Which of the following measures would potentially be most helpful in this scenario?

    (A) placing the patient on respiratory isolation
    (B) placing the patient on bodily secretion isolation
    (C) drawing blood only from arteries
    (D) placing the patient on reverse isolation

13. Common side effects of antibiotic therapy include which of the following?

    I. potential bone marrow suppression
    II. reduction in normal bacterial flora
    III. development of resistance to antibiotics
    (A) I and II
    (B) I and III
    (C) II and III
    (D) I, II, and III

14. Which cell secretes lymphokines (biological response modifiers)?

(A) segmented neutrophil
(B) band neutrophil
(C) T lymphocyte
(D) B lymphocyte

15. Which of the following is not a lymphokine?

(A) interferon
(B) interleukin
(C) GM-CSF (granulocyte-macrophage colony-stimulating factor)
(D) cyclosporine

16. Which antibody mediates allergic reactions?

(A) IgD
(B) IgM
(C) IgE
(D) IgG

17. Which is the most dominant antibody in adult life?

(A) IgA
(B) IgB
(C) IgC
(D) IgG

18. Which of the following would be given to provide passive immunity from accidental puncture with a needle contaminated with hepatitis?

(A) IgA
(B) IgB
(C) IgC
(D) IgG

19. The human immunodeficiency virus (HIV) works through inhibition of which aspect of the immune system?

(A) B-cell lymphocytes
(B) T-cell lymphocytes
(C) neutrophils
(D) complement

20. In a patient with pneumococcal pneumonia, which of the following classes of antibiotics may be useful in treatment?

I. penicillins
II. aminoglycosides
III. cephalosporins

    (A) I, II, and III
    (B) I and II
    (C) II and III
    (D) I and III

21. Which of the following agents is used to treat *Pneumocystis carinii* pneumonia?

    (A) Septra (Bactrim)
    (B) acyclovir
    (C) amphotericin B
    (D) vancomycin

Questions 22 and 23 refer to the following scenario.

A 64-year-old female is in your unit after a hepatic resection for cancer. During her second postoperative day, she complains of generalized discomfort with no change in incisional pain. She feels warm to the touch and her vital signs indicate the following:

blood pressure	96/56
pulse	115
respiratory rate	28
temperature	39° C

Lung sounds have scattered crackles throughout both lungs. Pulmonary artery catheter readings provide the following information:

CI	5.9
PA	28/14
PCWP	12
CVP	4
PaO_2	64
$PaCO_2$	35
pH	7.32
FIO_2	0.40

22. Based on the preceding information, which condition is possibly developing?

    (A) sepsis
    (B) CHF (congestive heart failure)
    (C) pneumonia
    (D) ARDS (adult respiratory distress syndrome)

23. Which treatment would most likely be instituted based on the preceding information?

    I. triple antibiotics
    II. amphotericin B
   III. fluid bolus

       (A) I, II
       (B) I, III
       (C) II, III
       (D) I, II, and III

24. Bone marrow failure occurring with leukemia can present with which of the following symptoms?

    I. bleeding
    II. increased risk of infection
   III. anemia

       (A) I, II, and III
       (B) I and II
       (C) II and III
       (D) I and III

25. In which organ system does much of the development of antibodies take place?

    (A) hepatic
    (B) respiratory
    (C) gastrointestinal
    (D) splenic

26. Which of the following is a/are common clinical presentation(s) of multiple myeloma?

    I. bone pain
    II. pathologic fractures
   III. stomatitis

       (A) I
       (B) III
       (C) II and III
       (D) I and II

27. Which immunologic disorder presents with Bence Jones proteinuria?

    (A) acute myelocytic leukemia
    (B) multiple myeloma
    (C) chronic myelocytic leukemia
    (D) lymphomas

Questions 28 and 29 refer to the following scenario.

A 37-year-old male is admitted to your unit for investigation of the cause of his hypotension. He has a history of weight loss, night sweats, and cervical lymph node enlargement. Laboratory data and vita signs reveal the following information:

blood pressure	88/60
pulse	118
respiratory rate	31
temperature	38.7
white blood cells	6,000
platelets	400,000

Reed-Sternberg cells are noted in the laboratory analysis.

28. Based on the preceding information, which condition is likely to be developing?

    (A) sepsis
    (B) multiple myeloma
    (C) Hodgkin's disease
    (D) acute lymphocytic leukemia

29. Which treatment modality or modalities could be employed in this patient?

    I. splenectomy
    II. radiation therapy
    III. chemotherapy
       (A) I and II
       (B) II and III
       (C) III
       (D) I, II, and III

30. Which phase of chronic myelocytic leukemia can resemble an acute leukemia?

    (A) blast crisis
    (B) recombinant phase
    (C) hematoporesis phase
    (D) myelosuppressive phase

Questions 31 and 32 refer to the following scenario.

A 27-year-old male with a history of homosexual behavior is admitted to your unit with shortness of breath, weight loss, and non productive cough. Current vital signs are:

blood pressure	118/74
pulse	114
respiratory rate	34
temperature	38.4

HIV (human immunodeficiency virus) serum testing is positive.

31. Based on the preceding information, which condition is likely to be present?

    (A) Kaposi's sarcoma
    (B) non-Hodgkin's lymphoma
    (C) Kleibsella pneumonia
    (D) *pneumocystis carinii* pneumonia

32. What is the likely cause for the shortness of breath?

    (A) noncardiogenic pulmonary edema
    (B) lymphocytic infiltration into the bronchi
    (C) V/Q disturbance from pneumonia
    (D) high P_aCO_2 levels

33. Which side effect of chemotherapy can affect nutritional status?

    (A) loss of serum proteins
    (B) stomatitis
    (C) increased oxygen consumption
    (D) loss of gastrointestinal function

34. Which condition occurs with the graft-versus-host response to transplanted bone marrow?

    (A) The body rejects the transplanted marrow.
    (B) The transplanted cells reject normal cells.
    (C) The donor cells mutate into abnormal host cells.
    (D) Both graft cells and normal cells reject each other.

35. At what point does spontaneous bleeding become a nursing concern in the patient receiving chemotheraphy?

(A) white blood cell count <3000/mm³
(B) fibrin split product level <400
(C) platelet count <20,000/mm³
(D) platelet count >50,000/mm³

36. Which is the first response in coagulation following trauma to a blood vessel?

(A) vasoconstriction
(B) platelet aggregation
(C) fibrin formation
(D) thrombin formation

37. Which electrolyte is an integral part of the coagulation process?

(A) sodium
(B) potassium
(C) magnesium
(D) calcium

Questions 38 and 39 refer to the following scenario.

A 41-year-old female is admitted to your unit with an exacerbation of chronic lympho-cytic leukemia. She states that she has had small amounts of vaginal bleeding. Ecchy-motic areas are noted on her arms and legs. Laboratory data reveal the following:

platelets	15,000/ mm³
white blood cells	4,000/ mm³
granulocytes	50%

38. Which of the following nursing measures should be employed on this pa-tient?

I. place on bleeding precautions
II. place on reverse isolation
III. avoid fresh plants and vegetables in the room
    (A) I
    (B) I and II
    (C) II and III
    (D) I, II, and III

39. Which treatment would most likely be ordered for this patient?

(A) platelet transfusions
(B) initiation of aerosolized pentamidine
(C) low-dose heparin therapy
(D) amphotericin B

40. Which of the following characterizes disseminated intravascular clotting?

(A) decreased prothrombin time
(B) increased levels of fibrinogen degradation products
(C) antithrombin formation
(D) platelet proliferation

41. A patient admitted with a diagnosis of pulmonary embolism is to receive a thrombolytic agent. Which of the following is NOT considered a thrombo-lytic medication?

(A) tissue plasminogen activator (tPA)
(B) urokinase
(C) streptokinase
(D) heparin

42. Which test is best employed to assess the effectiveness of heparin therapy?

(A) partial thromboplastin time (PTT)
(B) prothrombin time (PT)
(C) platelet levels
(D) bleeding time

43. The thrombolytic effect of plasmin is due to which action?

(A) preventing platelet aggregation
(B) blocking the intrinsic pathway
(C) breaking down of fibrin
(D) ionization of calcium

44. Which cell is characteristic of Hodgkin's disease?

(A) Kaposi
(B) Reed-Sternberg
(C) promyelocyte
(D) Stevens

45. Which lymphoma tends to progress along adjacent groups of lymph nodes, as opposed to skipping to noncontinuous groups?

(A) lymphocytic leukemia
(B) multiple myeloma
(C) non-Hodgkin's lymphoma
(D) Hodgkin's disease

Questions 46 and 47 refer to the following scenario.

A 35-year-old male is admitted to your unit with the diagnosis of Hodgkin's disease. He is admitted due to dyspnea, upper trunk edema, jugular venous distention, and cough.

46. Based on the preceding information, which condition is likely to be developing?

    (A) right ventricular failure
    (B) lymphocytic infiltration into the myocardium
    (C) superior vena caval syndrome
    (D) venous congestion secondary to splenic enlargement

47. Which treatment would most likely improve the symptoms?

    (A) diuretics
    (B) radiation therapy
    (C) administration of 5-FU (fluorouracil)
    (D) surgery to remove lymphatic obstructions

48. An 18-year-old black female is admitted to your unit with complaints of shortness of breath and severe joint pain. She has a history of sickle cell anemia. Measures to reduce patient discomfort should include which of the following?

    I. analgesics
    II. oxygen therapy
    III. normal saline fluid challenge

        (A) I and II
        (B) I and III
        (C) II and III
        (D) I, II, and III

49. Which of the following tests is used to diagnose a hemolytic transfusion reaction?

    (A) Coombs's test
    (B) PT (prothrombin time)
    (C) aPTT (activated partial thromboplastin time)
    (D) fibrinogen level

50. What is another name for Factor I?

    (A) fibrinogen
    (B) thrombin
    (C) prothrombin
    (D) thromboplastin

51. The extrinsic pathway for coagulation is initiated by which mechanism?

    (A) irregularity of the blood vessel wall
    (B) presence of atherosclerotic plaques causing increased turbulent blood flow
    (C) exposure to interstitial tissue following trauma to the blood vessel
    (D) introduction of an extrinsic substance into the blood

52. What is the cause of superior vena caval syndrome?

    (A) obstruction of the superior vena cava by thrombi
    (B) compression of the vena cava by enlarged lymph nodes
    (C) failure of the left and right heart due to lymphocytic infiltration
    (D) bronchial obstruction due to tumor growth

53. Advantages of having "normal flora" of bacteria on the skin include which of the following?

    I. They maintain the acidic pH of the skin.
    II. They compete successfully for nutrients with pathologic organisms.
    III. They produce oxygen for use by superficial cell layers.
       (A) I
       (B) II
       (C) I and II
       (D) II and III

54. Which antibody is naturally present in bodily secretions (e.g., saliva)?

    (A) IgG
    (B) IgQ
    (C) IgA
    (D) IgE

55. What is the primary purpose of the complement system?

    (A) to aid in the coagulation process
    (B) to assist antibodies in destroying antigens
    (C) to prevent the development of tumor cells
    (D) to act as scavengers to clear antigenic debris

56. The various components of the lymphatic drainage system combine to form a large thoracic duct. Where does the thoracic duct empty?

    (A) internal mammary artery
    (B) inferior vena cava
    (C) right atrium
    (D) left subclavian vein

57. What is the first stage in the coagulation process?

   (A) conversion of plasminogen to plasmin
   (B) conversion of fibrinogen to fibrin
   (C) activation of thrombin
   (D) activation of thromboplastin

58. Tissue plasminogen activator has potential advantages over streptokinase. What are these potential advantages?

   I. It is clot specific as opposed to systemic.
   II. It is less expensive.
   III. It has a shorter half-life.
      (A) I and II
      (B) I and III
      (C) II and III
      (D) I, II, and III

59. Nursing care of the patient receiving thrombolytic therapy includes which of the following?

   I. avoiding intramuscular injections
   II. using a soft toothbrush
   III. using oximetry rather than blood gas studies for SaO$_2$ determination
      (A) I and II
      (B) I and III
      (C) II and III
      (D) I, II, and III

60. Which component is primarily stored in the spleen?

   (A) platelets
   (B) neutrophils
   (C) lymphocytes
   (D) factor VIII

61. Which hormone is thought to regulate bone marrow production of platelets and red blood cells?

   (A) growth hormone
   (B) erythropoietin
   (C) thyroid-stimulating hormone
   (D) ACTH (adrenocorticotropic hormone)

CHAPTER 8 _____

Multisystem Organ Dysfunction Practice Exam

1. A 47-year-old male is admitted to your unit with the diagnosis of exacerabation of COPD (chronic obstructive pulmonary disease) with an acute bacterial pneumonia. His vital signs are as follows:

blood pressure	144/86
pulse	114
respiratory rate	28
temperature	39°C

Based on this information, what would you expect his baseline heart rate to be?

(A) 65
(B) 84
(C) 93
(D) 101

2. A 54-year-old female is admitted to your unit with the diagnosis "rule out sepsis of unknown origin." The most likely origin is a marked cellulitis involving most of her right leg. Her admitting white blood cell count is as follows:

white blood cells	21,000
segmented neutrophils	72%
banded neutrophils	9%
monocytes	5%
lymphocytes	13%
eosinophils	1%

Based on the white blood cell count, which of the values is/are abnormal (from a total count perspective)?

    I. segmented neutrophils
    II. banded neutrophils
    III. monocytes
    IV. lymphocytes

        (A) I and II
        (B) II and III
        (C) I, II, and III
        (D) IV

3. A 21-year-old male is in the intensive care unit following the development of acute respiratory failure after bone marrow transplantation. He has a white blood cell count of 1500 with segmented neutrophils of 30% and lymphocytes of 15%. His temperature is 37.5°C. Based on this information, does he meet the criteria for reverse isolation?

(A) Yes, his lymphocytes are only 15%.
(B) Yes, his total granulocyte count is probably less than $500/mm^3$.
(C) No, his total white blood cell count has not decreased to below $1000/mm^3$.
(D) No, he does not have a fever or active infection.

4. A blood culture report returns for a 73-year-old male who is in the intensive care unit for possible sepsis. The report states that he has *E. coli* (a gram-negative bacterium) in the blood. He currently is receiving gentamycin, imipenem, and ceftoxitin. Based on the report, what should be done about the antibiotic coverage?

(A) discontinue all drugs and start moxalactam
(B) maintain the current regime
(C) remove the imipenem and cefoxitin
(D) remove the gentamycin

Questions 5 and 6 refer to the following scenario.

A 69-year-old female is admitted to your unit with probable septic shock after sustaining a ruptured diverticulum in her large intestine. The following information is available:

blood pressure	80/52
pulse	121
respiratory rate	38
temperature	38°C
CO	8.9
CI	5.6

SI	46
PA	24/11
PCWP	8
CVP	2
PaO_2	78
$PaCO_2$	29
pH	7.32
HCO_3^-	16
lactate	5.1
SvO_2	81%
SpO_2	95%

5. Based on this information, which treatment(s) is/are likely to be implemented first?

    I. normal saline fluid bolus of 300 cc/30 min
   II. dobutamine at 5 mcg/kg per min
  III. administration of antipyretics
       (A) I and II
       (B) II and III
       (C) I and III
       (D) I, II, and III

6. Treatment with which of the following is most likely to reverse the effects of the sepsis?

   (A) HA-IA antibody
   (B) ibuprofen
   (C) dopamine
   (D) fluid bolus of either crystalloid or colloidal solutions

7. A 64-year-old female is in the intensive care unit with the diagnosis of possible sepsis secondary to a urinary tract infection. Upon admission she was markedly short of breath with an a/A (arterial/alveolar) ratio of 0.14, an FIO_2 of 0.80, and a PaO_2 of 72. She was intubated due to increased work of breathing. Shortly after admission, she became hypotensive and had a pulmonary artery catheter inserted to aid in management. Over the next two days, she was aggressively treated with normal saline fluid bolus (with a subsequent 10-kg weight gain), antibiotics, and dobutamine. Based on the following information, has the therapy been successful to this point?

	DAY 2	DAY 3	DAY 4
PaO_2	87	78	92
$PaCO_2$	35	32	37
pH	7.33	7.31	7.33
HCO_3^-	21	20	22
blood pressure	88/52	92/56	90/56
pulse	114	116	112
CO	8.6	8.9	9.3
CI	5.1	5.2	5.5
PA	42/32	46/35	39/33
PCWP	14	15	17
CVP	9	10	10
SvO_2	0.55	0.53	0.52
lactate	4	4.6	4.6

(A) yes, as illustrated by an increased CI
(B) yes, as illustrated by an increased PaO_2
(C) no, as illustrated by an unimproved SvO_2
(D) no, as illustrated by an increase in PCWP

Questions 8 and 9 refer to the following scenario.

A 64-year-old female is admitted to your unit following a house fire in which she suffered second-degree burns of both legs and her front torso. She is confused and cannot describe what happened. The following laboratory data are available:

PaO_2	88
$PaCO_2$	33
pH	7.36
HCO_3^-	21
FIO_2	0.28

8. Based on this information, how much of her body surface area was burned?

   (A) 15%
   (B) 27%
   (C) 39%
   (D) 55%

9. Which of the following would be considered initial therapies for this situation?

   I. mechanical ventilation
   II. administration of large volumes of lactated ringers
   III. silver sulfadiazine ointment

(A) I and II
(B) I and III
(C) II and III
(D) I, II, and III

10. Which of the following would be expected as part of the routine care of a patient who has a 40% second-degree burn?

I. topical antibiotics
II. wound debridement
III. increased caloric administration

(A) I and II
(B) I and III
(C) II and III
(D) I, II, and III

11. Which of the following are considered important for the increased survival of burn patients?

I. increased supply of cadaveric homografts
II. improved crystalloid resuscitation formulas
III. improved control of infections

(A) I and II
(B) I and III
(C) II and III
(D) I, II, and III

12. Which of the following is the most common reason for morbidity associated with burns?

(A) hypovolemia
(B) nutritional deficits
(C) sepsis
(D) acute respiratory failure

13. Monoclonal antibodies are of potential benefit in treating which of the following conditions?

I. sepsis
II. acute renal failure
III. ARDS (adult respiratory distress syndrome)

(A) I and II
(B) I and III
(C) II and III
(D) I, II, and III

Questions 14 and 15 refer to the following scenario.

A 26-year-old male was working in his basement with an acetylene torch when the flame started a fire in some nearby paper and wood. He states that the flame flashed toward his face but he quickly ran to the other side of the basement and got a fire extinguisher. The fire was not initially controlled by the extinguisher, so he ran outside. He is now admitted to your unit with second-degree upper torso and arm burns. In addition to the burns on his chest, his face is red with loss of facial hair. The following laboratory data are available:

pH	7.33
PaO_2	79
$PaCO_2$	29
HCO_3^-	21
FIO_2	0.30
SaO_2	0.83
CoHgb	0.16
MetHgb	0.01

14. Which of the following information would be suggestive of smoke inhalation in this patient?

    I. singed facial hair
    II. COHgb level of 16%
    III. MetHgb level of 1%
        (A) I and II
        (B) I and III
        (C) II and III
        (D) I, II, and III

15. Which treatment would most likely be given at this time?

    I. increased FIO_2 support
    II. paraffin soaks
    III. tracheobronchial suctioning
        (A) I and II
        (B) I and III
        (C) II and III
        (D) I, II, and III

16. In the patient with smoke inhalation, what is the most likely time period during which pulmonary complications may develop?

    (A) first 4 hours postinhalation
    (B) 4 to 18 hours postinhalation
    (C) 18 to 24 hours postinhalation
    (D) 24 to 48 hours postinhalation

17. Which of the following would be considered signs of carbon monoxide (COHgb) toxicity?

   I. parasympathetic stimulation
  II. confusion
 III. flushing of the face

     (A) I and II
     (B) I and III
     (C) II and III
     (D) I, II, and III

18. A 17-year-old male is admitted to your unit following an electric shock injury. His friends state that he was climbing a sign when a pole he was carrying touched a power line. He fell from the sign and was unresponsive. His friends immediately brought him to the emergency room. Based on the preceding description, which conditions could be anticipated to be present during the first 24 hours of intensive care unit admission?

   I. cardiac dysrhythmias
  II. rapid, systemic fluid shifts to third spaces
 III. pain in the burned area

     (A) I and II
     (B) I and III
     (C) II and III
     (D) I, II, and III

Questions 19 and 20 refer to the following scenario.

A 23-year-old male is admitted to your unit following a fire at his place of work, a paint factory. He has burns across his chest, arms, and upper legs. He is responsive to verbal stimuli and currently denies any pain. His vital signs are as follows:

blood pressure	104/62
pulse	134
respiratory rate	32

19. Based on the preceding information, which type of burn is likely to be present?

     (A) first-degree
     (B) partial-thickness
     (C) second-degree with loss of epithelial tissue
     (D) full-thickness

20. Which of the following would be the most likely initial therapy in this situation?

(A) administration of topical silver sulfidine
(B) administration of large volumes of intravenous lactated Ringer's
(C) administration of 100% oxygen
(D) placement of a Swan-Ganz catheter to assess fluid status

21. Which of the following is considered most useful for stabilizing hemodynamics in the immediate postburn resuscitation period?

(A) Hespan
(B) lactated Ringer's
(C) normal saline
(D) albumin

Questions 22 and 23 refer to the following scenario.

A 46-year-old male is in your unit following a fire in which the chair in which he was sitting was ignited by a cigarette. He is burned over 40% of his body (mostly back and lower extremities) with partial-thickness burns. It is now four days since he sustained the burns. He complains of pain in both legs, but particularly his right, which is covered with eschar.

22. Based on the preceding information, which method of pain relief would be the most appropriate?

I. escharotomy
II. intramuscular Demerol
III. intravenous morphine

(A) I and II
(B) I and III
(C) II and III
(D) I, II, and III

23. In this patient, what would be the advantage to performing an escharotomy?

I. pain relief
II. improvement in circulation
III. reduction in postburn scarring

(A) I and II
(B) I and III
(C) II and III
(D) I, II, and III

24. Which of the following organs is/are likely to be affected in multisystem organ dysfunction?

   I. liver
  II. kidney
 III. lungs

    (A) I and II
    (B) I and III
    (C) II and III
    (D) I, II, and III

25. The effects of tumor necrosing factor, leukotrienes, and thromboxane A$_2$ are similar in the systemic responses they initiate. Which of the following are consistent with the actions produced by these substances?

   I. vasoconstriction
  II. increasing cardiac ejection fraction
 III. promoting platelet aggregation

    (A) I and II
    (B) I and III
    (C) II and III
    (D) I, II, and III

26. A 19-year-old female is admitted to your unit after an argument with her parents. Her parents state that they found her in her room with an empty bottle of Tylenol on her nightstand. Which of the following is the initial treatment for an overdose of acetaminophen?

    (A) Ipecac
    (B) lavage and *N*-acetylcystine
    (C) dialysis
    (D) charcoal only

27. Which of the following are considered symptoms of aspirin poisoning?

   I. initial pH >7.45
  II. gastrointestinal bleeding
 III. late pH <7.35

    (A) I and II
    (B) I and III
    (C) II and III
    (D) I, II, and III

28. Tricyclic poisoning can produce lethal consequences from which of the following effects?

    (A) quinidine-like effects
    (B) neurologic injury secondary to seizures
    (C) parasympathetic stimulation
    (D) noncardiogenic pulmonary edema

29. Which of the following is a useful diagnostic sign when trying to determine the severity of a tricyclic poisoning attempt?

(A) presence of seizures
(B) tricyclic blood levels
(C) QRS complex narrowing
(D) widening pulse pressure

30. A burn involving the entire length of both lower extremities would constitute a burn over what percentage of the entire body?

(A) 9%
(B) 18%
(C) 36%
(D) 52%

31. A 20-year-old male is admitted to your unit following a suicide attempt after breaking up with his girl friend. He ingested an unknown drug or drugs and is currently combative but with a reduced level of consciousness. A large-bore nasogastric tube has been inserted in an attempt to lavage his stomach. Which of the following nursing actions should be initiated at this point?

I. protection against aspiration
II. intubation and mechanical ventilation
III. sedation to reduce the combativeness

(A) I
(B) II
(C) III
(D) I, II, and III

Questions 32 and 33 refer to the following scenario.

A 47-year-old male is admitted to the hospital following complaints of severe muscle weakness of the lower extremities. Neurologic examinations are negative, including MRI (magnetic resonance imaging) of the head and back. While on the medical floor, his level of consciousness changes and he is arousable only by deep stimuli. He requires intubation and mechanical ventilation. The following laboratory and vital sign information is available:

blood pressure	88/54
pulse	126
respiratory rate	24 (on assisted mandatory ventilation)
temperature	39°C
PaO$_2$	78

FIO_2	0.50
HCO_3^-	18
white blood cells	31,000
BUN	38
SGOT	433
pH	7.33
$PaCO_2$	32
Hgb	13
creatinine	2.6
SGPT	512
alkaline phosphatase	199

32. Based on this information, which condition is likely to be developing?

   (A) Guillain-Barré syndrome
   (B) ARDS
   (C) systemic inflammatory response syndrome
   (D) amyotrophic lateral sclerosis

33. Treatment for this condition is most likely to include which of the following?

   (A) increased intravenous fluids
   (B) plasmapheresis
   (C) dopamine
   (D) beta blockers, such as propranolol or esmolol

34. Which of the following are the most characteristic responses of the cardiovascular system to sepsis?

   I. increased ejection fraction
   II. increased cardiac output
   III. reduced systemic vascular resistance

   (A) I and II
   (B) I and III
   (C) II and III
   (D) I, II, and III

Questions 35 and 36 refer to the following scenario.

A 54-year-old female is in your unit following acute hepatic failure from hepatitis C, to be evaluated for a liver transplant and for management of a persistent fever (temperature >39°C). She becomes hypotensive (84/50) and tachycardic (130). A fiber optic pulmonary artery catheter is placed and reveals the following:

CO	12.9
CI	7.2
PA	30/12
PCWP	8
CVP	3
SvO_2	0.88

35. Based on the preceding information, which condition would explain her current clinical status?

(A) portal hypertension
(B) left ventricular failure
(C) hypovolemia secondary to loss of plasma proteins
(D) sepsis

36. Which of the following would explain the SvO_2 value of 0.88?

   I. increased oxygen consumption
  II. increased oxygen delivery
 III. pericapillary shunting

   (A) I and II
   (B) I and III
   (C) II and III
   (D) I, II, and III

37. Since the initial recognition of sepsis as a distinct disorder, particularly in the past 30 years, treatment has frequently been ineffective due to the inability to isolate a central mediating agent. Of the following, which has the most potential to be a central mediating agent in the development of sepsis?

(A) arachidonic acid
(B) monoclonal antibodies
(C) prostaglandins
(D) tumor necrosing factor

Questions 38 and 39 refer to the following scenario.

A 19-year-old soldier is brought to your hospital from a Middle Eastern country for treatment of an unidentifiable source of inflammation. He is restless and responsive only to deep pain and appears to be uncomfortable. His urine output has been 400 cc for the past 24 hours. The following physical and laboratory information is available:

blood pressure	100/54
pulse	133
respiratory rate	38

temperature	39.5°C
white blood cells	19,300
red blood cells	3,500,300
Hgb	11
Hct	32
Na^+	155
K^+	3.9
Cl^-	111
HCO_3^-	26
urinary Na^+	9
urinary osmolality	878

38. Based on the preceding information, the physician wants to start a fluid bolus with 500 cc of normal saline. Which of the following findings support this decision?

    I. red blood cell count of 3,500,300
    II. Na^+ level of 155
    III. clinical picture of systemic inflammation

        (A) I and II
        (B) I and III
        (C) II and III
        (D) I, II, and III

39. Given an unknown source of inflammation, which of the following therapies would most likely be prescribed?

    I. aminoglycosides (e.g., gentamicin)
    II. antiinflammatory agents (e. g., methylprednisolone)
    III. cephalosporins (e.g., cefoxitine)

        (A) I and II
        (B) I and III
        (C) II and III
        (D) I, II, and III

Questions 40 and 41 refer to the following scenario.

A 38-year-old female is in your unit with a fever of unknown origin. She became acutely short of breath on the step-down floor and was transferred to the unit. She required intubation and mechanical ventilation when her shortness of breath could not be relieved. Her present ventilator settings are AMV (assist/control), rate 12 (total rate 34), tidal volume 700 cc, FIO_2 0.70. Her mental status is confused and she is restless and pulling at her tubes, requiring her to be restrained. She currently has the following vital signs and laboratory data:

blood pressure	136/82
pulse	127
respiratory rate	34
temperature	38.8°C
PaO_2	65
$PaCO_2$	34
pH	7.31
HCO_3^-	17

40. One of your fellow nurses states that, in systemic inflammatory responses like the preceding situation, oxygen consumption and energy requirements are increased. Another nurse says that that is not always true, that only in some instances are energy requirements increased. Which of the preceding pieces of information suggests that this patient has increased energy expenditure and oxygen consumption?

   I. respiratory rate of 34
   II. PaO_2 of 65
   III. temperature of 38.8°C
       (A) I and II
       (B) I and III
       (C) II and III
       (D) I, II, and III

41. Which of the following therapies would be designed to help reduce the energy expenditure in this patient?

   I. changing to IMV (intermittent mandatory ventilation) from AMV
   II. administering sedation, such as a benzodiazepem (e.g., 1 to 2 mg Versed)
   III. administering an antipyretic, such as acetaminophen (Tylenol)
       (A) I and II
       (B) I and III
       (C) II and III
       (D) I, II, and III

Questions 42 and 43 refer to the following scenario.

A 76-year-old male on postoperative day 5 following a colon resection for a bowel obstruction develops a fever of 39°C. He has no overt signs of infection. During the evening he becomes hypotensive and is transferred to your unit. A pulmonary artery catheter is placed and the following information is available:

blood pressure	84/50
pulse	116
respiratory rate	29

temperature	39°C
PaO_2	88
FIO_2	0.50
PA	20/8
PCWP	5
CO	9.1
CI	6.0
SvO_2	0.81
PvO_2	50

Based on this information, the physician states that she believes the symptoms are consistent with the diagnosis of sepsis.

42. Which of the following clinical signs are consistent with the diagnosis of sepsis?

    I. SvO_2 of 0.81
    II. CI of 6.0
    III. PCWP of 5
        (A) I and II
        (B) I and III
        (C) II and III
        (D) I, II, and III

43. Which of the following would be indications of an improvement in the septic condition?

    (A) decrease in PCWP
    (B) increase in PaO_2
    (C) decrease in SvO_2
    (D) increase in CI

44. Which of the following are the two most common sources of infection in the critically ill population?

    I. urinary tract infection
    II. respiratory system infection
    III. central nervous system infection
        (A) I and II
        (B) I and III
        (C) II and III
        (D) they are all equal in the incidence of infections

Comprehensive Practice Exam—1

In this edition, you have two practice exams to utilize in your preparation for the CCRN exam. You may use them in any way you like, however, you might want to take the first exam (Chapter 9) and review the questions you missed. Then, after further study, you could take the second exam (Chapter 10).

The practice of taking exams as an exercise, should help you improve your score on the CCRN exam. Remember, no practice exam will exactly simulate the actual CCRN exam. However, the exams you are seeing here have been prepared by clinicians who have taken the CCRN exam and are familiar with the format and general type of questions asked. Good luck as you take these last two exams. We sincerely hope that they will help you in your preparation for the CCRN exam.

Questions 1 and 2 refer to the following scenario.

A 63-year-old male is admitted to your unit with an anterior wall MI (myocardial infarction). His blood pressure is 92/56 with a heart rate of 102. During your discussion with the physician, the question arises of whether treatment to increase the blood pressure should be started. One drug suggested is dopamime.

1. What would be the effect of adding a vasopressor such as dopamine?

    (A) decrease CVP (central venous pressure) and myocardial oxygen consumption
    (B) increase systemic vascular resistance and myocardial oxygen consumption
    (C) increase PCWP (pulmonary capillary wedge pressure) and decrease myocardial oxygen consumption
    (D) increase cardiac output and decrease PCWP

2. How would you make a determination of whether the blood pressure is low enough to be of clinical concern?

   I. assess the cardiac output
   II. measure blood gases for a PaO_2 value
   III. assess level of consciousness

   (A) I and II
   (B) I and III
   (C) II and III
   (D) I, II, and III

Questions 3 and 4 refer to the following scenario.

A 57-year-old male is admitted to your unit with the complaint of epigastric discomfort. He says that he took "a couple of swigs of Maalox" but the discomfort has not gone away. The pain has been present for about the past four hours. An admission ECG (electrocardiogram) has been obtained and is shown below.

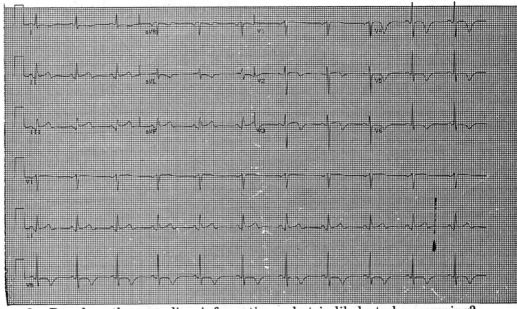

3. Based on the preceding information, what is likely to be occurring?

   (A) anterior myocardial ischemia
   (B) no ECG abnormality is present
   (C) inferior wall injury pattern
   (D) pericarditis

4. Which therapy is most likely to resolve the cause of this condition?

(A) thrombolytic therapy
(B) nitroglycerine
(C) H_2 blocker
(D) oxygen therapy

Questions 5 and 6 refer to the following scenario.

A 62-year-old male is admitted to your unit with the symptoms of shortness of breath and orthopnea. He has an S_3 heart sound, bilateral dependent pulmonary crackles, and distended jugular veins. His 12-lead ECG shows no ST segment changes, although Q waves are present in II, III, and aVF. A pulmonary artery catheter is placed and reveals the following information:

blood pressure	104/68
pulse	110
PA	38/24
PCWP	22
CVP	14
CO	4.1
CI	2.2

5. Based on the preceding information, which condition is likely to be developing?

(A) cardiogenic shock
(B) hypovolemic shock
(C) biventricular (congestive) failure
(D) pulmonary hypertension secondary to right ventricular failure

6. Which of the following would be an appropriate treatment choice?

(A) dobutamine
(B) dopamine
(C) normal saline fluid bolus
(D) diltiazem

7. A physician is attempting to insert a central line and states that the internal jugular approach is superior since there is less chance of causing a pneumothorax. If you were to listen to the lung after the insertion attempt to assess for a pneumothorax, where would be the best location to hear the superior border of the lung?

(A) slightly above the clavicle
(B) slightly below the clavicle
(C) at the second ICS (intercostal space)
(D) near the fourth ICS

Questions 8 and 9 refer to the following scenario.

A 28-year-old male is in the intensive care unit following a fall from a one-story rooftop three days ago. At the time he suffered a fractured left femur and right humerus. No neurologic or chest trauma occurred. He has large contusions over his right lower flank. During the last 24 hours, his urine output has fallen to 300 cc. He has had a 1-lb increase in weight since yesterday. Vital signs are as follows:

blood pressure	140/86
pulse	106
respiratory rate	25
temperature	38.3°C

Laboratory studies reveal the following information:

Na^+	136
K^+	4.3
Cl^-	103
HCO_3^-	22
creatinine	2.8
BUN	36
urinary Na^+	72
urinary osmolality	302

8. Based on the preceding information, which condition is likely to be developing?

   (A) prerenal azotemia
   (B) acute tubular necrosis
   (C) postrenal failure
   (D) hypovolemic induced prerenal failure

9. What would the primary treatment include at this point?

   (A) fluid bolus
   (B) dialysis
   (C) diuretics
   (D) CAVHD (continuous arterial/venous hemodialysis)

10. Elevations in intracranial pressure can be caused by which of the following?

   (A) hypovolemia
   (B) hypercarbia
   (C) hyperventilation
   (D) hypotension

11. Interpret the following ECG rhythm strip.

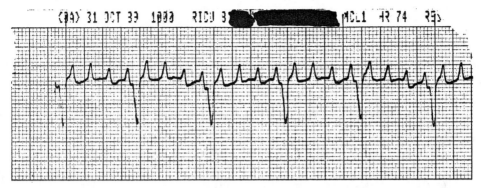

(A) atrial tachycardia with block
(B) third-degree block
(C) second-degree block, type I
(D) atrial flutter with block

Questions 12 and 13 refer to the following scenario.

Early in the afternoon, another nurse asks you to examine her patient since she "looks different" than earlier and her blood pressure is lower than that recorded that morning. When you examine the patient, you notice that her right breast is larger than her left. Upon auscultation of her chest, you notice diminished breath sounds on the right and distant heart sounds. The nurse states that no new procedures have been performed, although a central line was inserted earlier in the day. The patient is confused, although this has been noted throughout her admission. She is now more restless, however, with her pulse oximeter displaying a value of 0.94 on 5 LPM of nasal oxygen. Her vital signs are as follows:

blood pressure	98/62
pulse	107
respiratory rate	31
temperature	36.8°C

12. Based on the preceding information, which condition is likely to be developing?

(A) pericardial tamponade
(B) sepsis
(C) pneumomediastinum
(D) right-side pneumothorax

13. Which therapy should be instituted to treat the condition?

    (A) pericardiocentesis
    (B) anterior chest tube
    (C) mediastinal chest tube
    (D) No therapy is necessary; the patient requires only observation at this time.

14. Reverse isolation is frequently initiated when which immunologic finding is noted?

    (A) lymphocyte count of 1500 to 3000/mm³
    (B) temperature elevation of 104°F
    (C) left-sided shift in the differential
    (D) granulocyte count of less than 500/mm³

Questions 15 and 16 refer to the following scenario.

A 34-year-old male is in your unit following changes in behavior at home. His wife states that he has been on a liquid diet and has been drinking 5 L of water a day in an attempt to lose weight. He has generally been in good health and has not recently been to a physician. She states that her husband has had to "go to the bathroom" more often since the diet started. His vital signs and laboratory data are listed below.

blood pressure	148/88
pulse	104
respiratory rate	26
temperature	37.3
Na^+	108
K^+	3.8
Cl^-	78
HCO_3^-	21
osmolality	264

15. Based on the preceding information, which condition is likely to be developing?

    (A) malnutrition
    (B) acute high-output renal failure
    (C) hypoosmolality-induced CNS (central nervous system) deterioration
    (D) hyponatremia-induced behavior changes

16. Which therapy should be initiated to treat this condition?

    (A) increased calories
    (B) diuretics
    (C) 1000 cc of 3% NaCl
    (D) vasopressin

17. Which of the following is used in clinical settings to estimate preload of the left ventricle?

    (A) CVP (central venous pressure)
    (B) systemic vascular resistance
    (C) MAP (mean arterial pressure)
    (D) PCWP (pulmonary capillary wedge pressure)

Questions 18 and 19 refer to the following scenario.

A 21-year-old male college student is admitted to your unit following a fall from a tree during a prank. He is alert and oriented and complains of shortness of breath and chest pain on the right. He states that he landed on his right chest, a point confirmed by other witnesses. On physical examination, he has no overt trauma to the chest, breath sounds are diminished on the right, and the trachea is deviated to the left. His ECG shows nonspecific ST changes and analysis of his blood gases reveals the following:

pH	7.48
$PaCO_2$	28
PaO_2	69
FIO_2	room air

18. Based on the preceding information, which condition is developing?

    (A) myocardial contusion
    (B) open pneumothorax
    (C) tension pneumothorax
    (D) tracheal rupture

19. Which treatment would be indicated for his condition?

    (A) open thoracotomy
    (B) chest tube insertion
    (C) emergent tracheostomy
    (D) pericardiocentesis

20. A 49-year-old male is in your unit following surgery for colon cancer. During your shift, he develops a fever (39°C) and an increased white blood cell count (15,000). Levels of which of the following will be elevated if this is a new infection?

    (A) lymphocytes
    (B) monocytes
    (C) neutrophils
    (D) antibodies

Questions 21 and 22 refer to the following scenario.

A 24-year-old male is admitted to your unit after developing severe muscle weakness. His condition has been related to excessive ingestion of black licorice. His vital signs and electrolyte report are as follows:

blood pressure	134/72
pulse	106
respiratory rate	24
temperature	37°C
Na^+	147
K^+	1.8
Cl^-	116
HCO_3^-	22

21. Based on the preceding information, which other clinical symptoms may be present in this person?

    I. tall peaked T waves on the ECG
    II. PVCs (premature ventricular contractions) on the ECG
    III. behavioral changes
        (A) I
        (B) I and III
        (C) II
        (D) II and III

22. Which therapy would be useful in treating this condition?

    (A) diuretics
    (B) sodium bicarbonate ($NaHCO_3$)
    (C) potassium chloride (KCl)
    (D) sodium chloride (NaCl) fluid bolus

23. A 48-year-old male is admitted to your unit following an episode of hemetemesis. He states that he has had three such episodes prior to coming to the hospital. Based on this information, he is likely to be in a hypovolemic state and to experience loss of stroke volume. Which of the following components of cardiac output will compensate for the loss of stroke volume?

    (A) heart rate
    (B) systemic vascular resistance
    (C) MAP (mean arterial pressure)
    (D) CVP (central venous pressure)

24. A compensated respiratory acidosis would demonstrate which two blood gas findings?

(A) elevated $PaCO_2$ and decreased HCO_3^-
(B) decreased $PaCO_2$ and PaO_2
(C) increased HCO_3^- and decreased $PaCO_2$
(D) increased $PaCO_2$ and HCO_3^-

25. Upon performing an abdominal examination on your patient, you notice tympanic sounds upon percussing the left lower quadrant. Which sounds should be heard in the left lower quadrant under normal circumstances?

(A) tympanic
(B) resonant
(C) dull
(D) flat

26. A 55-year-old male has a history of systemic hypertension. Which of the following ECG changes are characteristic of chronic hypertension with left ventricular hypertrophy?

(A) large Q waves in II, III, and aVF
(B) a reversed R:S ratio in lead V_1
(C) large S waves in V_1 and large R waves in V_5
(D) ST segment elevation in all precordial leads

Questions 27 and 28 are based on the following scenario.

A 61-year-old female is admitted to your unit at 1500 after repair of an abdominal aortic aneurysm. Her admission vital signs and hemodynamics are stable and within normal limits. At 2000, she complains of abdominal discomfort unrelated to incisional pain. Her breath sounds are clear, her skin is cool, and she has no shortness of breath. The following hemodynamic information is available:

blood pressure	100/60
pulse	112
PA	23/10
PCWP	6
CVP	2
CO	3.6
CI	2.0

27. Based on the preceding information, which condition is likely to be developing?

(A) left ventricular failure
(B) hypovolemia
(C) sepsis
(D) cardiogenic shock

28. Which initial treatment would best support her hemodynamic function?

(A) Lasix
(B) dobutamine
(C) normal saline bolus
(D) dopamine

29. The primary effects of sepsis include which of the following?

I. increased coagulation tendencies
II. vasoconstriction at the capillary level
III. alteration of capillary permeability

(A) I and II
(B) I and III
(C) II and III
(D) I, II, and III

Questions 30 and 31 refer to the following scenario.

A 24-year-old male is in your unit following a fight in which he received multiple stab wounds to his chest and abdomen. He is now in his fourth postoperative day and is being considered for transfer to the floor. On your shift, he develops a temperature of 38.6°C. He complains of increasing shortness of breath and you note that his pulse oximeter reading has decreased from 0.99 to 0.92 in the last hour. A chest x ray reveals widespread infiltrates in both lungs. He is alert and oriented, although he states that he feels "tired." His heart rate is 122 (up from 84) and his respiratory rate is 33 (up from 18). Blood gas analysis and laboratory data reveal the following:

pH	7.33
$PaCO_2$	30
PaO_2	67
HCO_3^-	18
FIO_2	0.50
white blood cells	15,400
segmented neutrophils	66
lymphocytes	19
monocytes	11
other	4

30. Based on the preceding information, which condition is likely to be developing?

(A) recurrent atelectasis
(B) mucous plugging
(C) sepsis
(D) generalized pneumonia

31. Which therapy is most likely to be effective in improving the clinical situation?

(A) oxygen therapy
(B) postural drainage and percussion
(C) aerosol therapy
(D) antibiotic administration

Questions 32 and 33 refer to the following scenario.

A 59-year-old male is admitted to your unit with chest pain for the last hour. It is unrelieved by rest or nitroglycerine. He is short of breath and mildly orthopneic. A 12-lead ECG indicates ST segment elevation in V_1 through V_4 with ST segment depression in II, III, and aVF. No Q waves are present.

32. Based on the preceding symptoms and ECG findings, which condition is likely to be developing?

(A) Prinzmetal's angina
(B) inferior MI (myocardial infarction)
(C) CHF (congestive heart failure); no MI can be occuring due to the absence of Q waves
(D) anterior MI

33. Which of the following treatments is most likely to prevent further myocardial damage?

(A) TPA (tissue plasminogen activator)
(B) nitroglycerine (TNG)
(C) dobutamine
(D) Lasix

Questions 34 and 35 refer to the following scenario.

A thin, 64-year-old female was admitted to your unit with severe shortness of breath accompanying her diagnosis of COPD (chronic obstructive pulmonary disease). She had complained of gradually increasing shortness of breath over the past two days. Her oral tempature is 38°C. Her chest x ray indicates a consolidation in the left lower lobe. She has the following blood gas values:

pH	7.36
PaO_2	52
$PaCO_2$	33
HCO_3^-	26
FIO_2	0.40

34. Based on the preceding information, which condition is likely to be developing?

    (A) acute pulmonary oxygenation failure
    (B) acute pulmonary oxygenation and ventilation failure
    (C) acute and chronic ventilation failure
    (D) chronic ventilation failure

35. Treatment of this condition would center on which of the following areas?

    (A) intubation and mechanical ventilation
    (B) PEEP (positive end expiratory pressure) or CPAP (continuous positive airway pressure) therapy
    (C) antibiotic and oxygen therapy
    (D) bronchodilator and IPPB (intermittent positive pressure, breathing) treatment

36. A sudden increase in pain in a patient admitted with duodenal ulcers may indicate that which condition is developing?

    (A) increase in bleeding
    (B) spreading of the ulcer to the pain-sensitive gastrum
    (C) perforation of the ulcer
    (D) pancreatic ulcer formation

Questions 37 and 38 refer to the following scenario.

A 73-year-old female in previously good health is admitted to your unit with complaints of intermittent chest pain for the past six hours. The chest pain is unrelated to activity, although it worsens if she "moves around during a spell." She has no shortness of breath but does complain of "swelling" of her feet during the day. A 12-lead ECG demonstrates ST segment depression in I, aVL, V_5, and V_6. No Q waves exist in the ECG. Her finger oximeter reveals an SaO_2 value of 0.96 on room air.

37. Based on the preceding information, which condition is likely to be developing?

    (A) pulmonary emboli
    (B) angina
    (C) anterior MI (myocardial infarction)
    (D) left ventricular failure

38. Which treatment should be initially started for this condition?

    (A) Lasix
    (B) dobutamine
    (C) nitroglycerine
    (D) nifedipine

Questions 39 and 40 refer to the following scenario.

A 56-year-old, slightly overweight male is admitted to your unit with exacerbation of COPD (chronic obstructive pulmonary disease). A physical examination reveals that he is short of breath, is alert and oriented, and demonstrates inspiratory crackles and expiratory wheezes. He has circumoral cyanosis and pedal edema. Analysis of his blood gases reveals the following:

pH	7.34
PaO_2	52
$PaCO_2$	73
HCO_3^-	40
FIO_2	room air

39. Based on the preceding information, which underlying form of COPD is most likely to be present in this patient?

    (A) acute bronchitis
    (B) emphysema
    (C) chronic asthma
    (D) chronic bronchitis

40. Which initial form of treatment is indicated in this patient?

    (A) judicious oxygen therapy
    (B) intubation and mechanical ventilation
    (C) PEEP (positive end expiratory pressure) or CPAP (continuous positive airway pressure)
    (D) diuretic therapy

41. Clinical symptoms of sepsis may vary, depending on the stage. Which of the following are considered common septic symptoms?

    I. hypothermia
    II. hyperthermia
    III. bradycardia

    (A) I and II
    (B) I and III
    (C) II and III
    (D) I, II, and III

Questions 42 and 43 refer to the following scenario.

A 68-year-old male is admitted to your unit with severe abdominal pain radiating to the back. The pain does not subside with rest or position change. Oxygen therapy and sublingual nitroglycerine do not relieve the pain. He is diaphoretic with cool skin, but has no difficulty breathing. Breath sounds are clear. S_1 and S_2 are heard clearly and are the only heart sounds. His blood pressure is 172/100, pulse 114. His ECG shows a 1-mm ST depression in V_1.

42. Based on the preceding information, which condition is likely to be developing?

(A) anterior MI (myocardial infarction)
(B) recalcitrant angina
(C) pulmonary emboli
(D) abdominal aortic aneurysm

43. Which treatment would most likely be employed in this patient?

(A) abdominal aortic aneurysm repair
(B) thrombolytic therapy
(C) intravenous nitroglycerine
(D) sedation

44. The "high airway pressure" alarm on the ventilator is activated, indicating a worsening of the patient's pulmonary dynamic compliance. Which of the following are potential reasons for the pulmonary dynamic compliance to worsen?

I. airway secretions
II. mucous plugging
III. increased lung water

    (A) I and II
    (B) I and III
    (C) II and III
    (D) I, II, and III

45. Initial symptoms of colon cancer typically include which of the following?

(A) epigastric cramping
(B) anorexia
(C) rectal bleeding
(D) ascites

46. A 20-year-old male is in your unit with a severe head injury following a motor vehicle accident. He has been in the unit for 24 hours. On your shift, his ICP (intracranial pressure) changes from 14 to 31. The physician states that the volume-pressure relationship in the brain may have reached a critical point. Which of the following statements best describes the volume-pressure relationship within the skull when brain compliance is decreased?

(A) Large increases in volume will cause small pressure increases.
(B) Large increases in pressure will cause small volume increases.
(C) Small increases in volume will cause small pressure increases.
(D) Small increases in volume will cause large pressure increases.

47. Maintaining the $PaCO_2$ at 25 to 30 mm Hg can be helpful in managing ICP (intracranial pressure) due to its effect on which of the mechanisms listed below?

(A) cerebral blood flow
(B) cerebral tissue edema
(C) production of CSF (cerebrospinal fluid)
(D) systemic blood pressure

48. A 50-year-old female returns from cardiac catheterization with a report of a complete obstruction of the left anterior descending artery. Which condition may result from this situation?

(A) superior vena caval syndrome
(B) anterior MI (myocardial infarction)
(C) inferior MI
(D) posterior MI

49. A patient admitted with the diagnosis of cardiogenic shock requires mechanical ventilation. Which form of ventilation would be most appropriate to reduce his work of breathing?

(A) IMV (intermittent mandatory ventilation)
(B) pressure support ventilation
(C) assist/control ventilation
(D) PEEP (positive end expiratory pressure)

Questions 50 and 51 refer to the following scenario.

A 62-year-old female is in the intensive care unit following a cardiac arrest two days ago. She is responsive only to painful stimuli. Vital signs include a blood pressure of 86/56 and a pulse of 110. She is receiving mechanical ventilation on assist control of 10 bpm (with no spontaneous breathing), tidal volume 750 cc, FIO_2 0.40. Her urine output has decreased over the past 24 hours to 150 cc. The latest hemodynamic data are as follows:

PA	23/8
PCWP	7
CVP	2
CO	3.7
CI	2.2

Laboratory data are listed below:

	SERUM	URINE
Na+	146	11
K+	3.6	
osmolality	288	1090
Cl-	96	
creatinine	3	
BUN	60	

50. Based on the preceding information, which condition is likely to be developing?

(A) hypovolemic prerenal azotemia
(B) acute tubular necrosis
(C) postrenal failure secondary to ureteral obstruction
(D) hypernatremia-induced renal failure

51. Which of the following treatments would be indicated at this point?

(A) diuretics
(B) fluid bolus
(C) norepinephrine (Levophed)
(D) dobutamine

52. A 78-year-old female is admitted from the emergency room after being found unresponsive at home. She is hypotensive and requires mechanical ventilation to support her breathing. A pulmonary artery catheter is inserted to assist in identifying her primary problem. The inital ECG is unremarkable. At 0500, the physician requests that dobutamine administration be started to improve her hemodynamics. In the readings to be obtained at 0600, which parameters would be expected if the dobutamine has been effective?

	0400	0500
blood pressure	106/66	104/62
pulse	111	105
CI	2.4	2.5
PA	34/23	32/21
PCWP	21	17
CVP	12	11

I. decreased pulmonary capillary wedge pressure
II. increased stroke volume
III. increased pulmonary artery pressure

(A) I and II
(B) I and III
(C) II and III
(D) I, II, and III

53. A 59-year-old male is in your unit with pulmonary edema from an MI (myocardial infarction). He currently is on assist/control ventilation and is triggering the ventilator for a total rate of 32. In order to read his PCWP (pulmonary capillary wedge pressure) tracing accurately and avoid respiratory artifact, where is the best location on the waveform?

(A) end inspiration
(B) end expiration
(C) initial expiration
(D) initial inspiration

Questions 54 and 55 refer to the following scenario.

A 32-year-old female is admitted to your unit following a house fire in which she was rescued after losing consciousness. She has a 30% burn, with most of the burns on her back and legs.

54. Upon admission to the unit, which therapies are most likely to be initiated?

I. aggressive fluid resuscitation
II. topical antimicrobial agents (e.g., Silvadene)
III. occlusive dry dressings
(A) I and II
(B) I and III
(C) II and III
(D) I, II, and III

55. Which test would be performed to assess the extent of her smoke inhalation?

(A) chest x ray
(B) measurement of carboxyhemoglobin level
(C) arterial blood gas analysis
(D) ventilation/perfusion lung scan

56. Which findings, due to increased dead space, are almost always present in a patient with a pulmonary embolism?

(A) tachypnea and tachycardia
(B) hyperventilation and hypercarbia
(C) decreased pH and hypoxemia
(D) increased respiratory rate and decreased tidal volume

Questions 57 and 58 refer to the following scenario.

A 61-year-old female is admitted to your unit from her physician's office for possible dehydration. The dehydration is the result of anorexia and low fluid intake during the last several days due to a "cold." The family states that she has shown behavioral changes and has been extremely lethargic during the last two days. She has lost 10 lb in the last week, probably due to an increased urine output, based on family history. Laboratory results reveal the following information:

Na^+	153
K^+	3.5
Cl^-	114
HCO_3^-	20
osmolality	367
glucose	1020

57. Based on the preceding information, which condition is present?

    (A) insulin reaction
    (B) DKA (diabetic ketoacidosis)
    (C) thyroid storm
    (D) HHNK (hyperosmolar, hyperglycemic, nonketotic) coma

58. Treatment for this condition would center on which therapy?

    (A) glucose bolus (50 cc of $D_{50}W$)
    (B) insulin bolus and normal saline
    (C) insulin drip without bolus
    (D) thyroxine and glucocorticoids

59. A 62-year-old male is admitted to your unit with possible pericarditis. If pericarditis is present, which of the following symptoms would be present?

    (A) S_3 or gallop rhythm
    (B) split S_2
    (C) pleural friction rub worsening on inspiration
    (D) ST segment elevation in most leads of the 12-lead ECG

60. Given the following blood gas values, identify which condition is present.

pH	7.23
PaO_2	85
$PaCO_2$	26
HCO_3^-	16

(A) respiratory alkalosis alone
(B) metabolic acidosis alone
(C) combined respiratory and metabolic acidosis
(D) respiratory alkalosis and metabolic acidosis

61. A 59-year-old female with a history of alcoholism is admitted to your unit after being found unresponsive. During the next 24 hours, she develops decreased blood flow to her distal extremities, manifested by discoloration of her hands and feet. The physician believes that DIC (disseminated intravascular clotting) may be taking place. Which of the following tests may help confirm that DIC is present?

(A) measurment of platelet levels
(B) determination of bleeding time
(C) measurment of fibrinogen degradation product levels
(D) determination of plasminogen to plasmin converting time

62. Immunoglobulins are derived from which component of the white blood cell differential?

(A) B-cell lymphocytes
(B) T-cell lymphocytes
(C) segmented neutrophils
(D) monocytes

63. Hyperglycemia frequently presents with all of the following physical symptoms but one. Which of the following symptoms does NOT characterize hyperglycemic reactions?

(A) cool skin
(B) increased respirations
(C) increased urine output
(D) tachycardia

64. The PCWP (pulmonary capillary wedge pressure) estimates which of the following hemodynamic parameters?

(A) left ventricular end diastolic pressure
(B) mean pulmonary artery pressure
(C) cardiac output
(D) left ventricular end systolic pressure

65. Which of the following is the LEAST accurate estimate of intrapulmonary shunting?

(A) A-a (alveolar-arterial) gradient
(B) a/A (arterial-alveolar) ratio
(C) respiratory index
(D) PaO_2/FIO_2 ratio

66. Major complications of pancreatic surgery include which of the following?

(A) overproduction of insulin
(B) stimulation of glucagon production
(C) inhibition of trypsin production
(D) leakage of digestive enzymes into the pancreas

67. A 73-year-old male with a history of CHF (congestive heart failure) is placed on an afterload-reducing drug. Which of the following measures would be used to assess the effectiveness of afterload reduction?

(A) PCWP (pulmonary capillary wedge pressure)
(B) CVP (central venous pressure)
(C) SVR (systemic vascular resistance)
(D) MAP (mean arterial pressure)

68. A 33-year-old female is admitted with the diagnosis of possible adrenal cortical tumor. Levels of which of the following hormones would NOT likely be altered in this situation?

(A) cortisol
(B) epinephrine
(C) aldosterone
(D) androgens

69. While interpreting a pulmonary capillary wedge pressure, you note the presence of giant V waves. Which of the following conditions can produce giant V waves on a hemodynamic waveform?

   I. mitral regurgitation
  II. left bundle branch block
 III. noncompliant left atrium

(A) I and II
(B) I and III
(C) II and III
(D) I, II, and III

70. A 71-year-old male with the diagnosis of chronic lung disease has cyanosis of the nailbeds. How can a patient have cyanosis and still have adequate oxygen transport?

(A) He can if the oxyhemoglobin curve is shifted to the left.
(B) He can if the hemoglobin and cardiac output are adequate.
(C) He can if the FIO_2 is high enough to raise CaO_2 values.
(D) Oxygen transport cannot be adequate with the presence of cyanosis.

71. A 54-year-old female is in your unit with acute tubular necrosis. As a result of the acute renal failure, she has developed hyperkalemia. She does not yet have vascular access for dialysis to be initiated. Which of the following therapies could be used to treat the hyperkalemia prior to the use of dialysis?

   I. ammonium chloride resin
  II. kayexalate
 III. glucose insulin infusion

   (A) I and II
   (B) I and III
   (C) II and III
   (D) I, II, and III

Questions 72 and 73 refer to the following scenario.

A 23-year-old male is in the intensive care unit following a closed head injury from a fight. During the second day of hospitalization, he develops a severe thirst and is consuming 1000 cc of water per shift. Urine output is 2000 cc per shift. An electrolyte analysis is obtained and reveals the following data:

Na^+	150
K^+	3.6
Cl^-	118
HCO_3^-	23
osmolality	324
glucose	178
urinary osmolality	304
urinary Na^+	61

72. Based on the preceding information, which condition is developing?

   (A) hyperosmolar, nonketotic acidosis
   (B) diabetes insipidus
   (C) diabetic ketoacidosis
   (D) thyroid storm

73. Which treatment would be indicated for this condition?

(A) insulin-glucose infusion
(B) DDAVP (Desmopressin acetate)
(C) Hageman factor in intravenous form
(D) diuretics

Questions 74 and 75 refer to the following scenario.

A 49-year-old female is admitted to your unit with a history of primary pulmonary hypertension. Her pulmonary artery blood pressure is 70/46. She complains of a marked decrease in exercise capability and persistent shortness of breath. Her 12-lead ECG shows the following: 5-mm R wave in V_1 and V_2, 4-mm S wave in V_1. She has small Q waves in leads II, III, and aVF. Her underlying rhythm is sinus tachycardia.

74. Based on the preceding information, which condition is likely to be present?

(A) pulmonary edema
(B) non–Q wave anterior-inferior MI (myocardial infarction)
(C) left ventricular hypertrophy
(D) right ventricular hypertrophy

75. Treatment for this condition would most likely include which of the following?

I. Lasix
II. oxygen therapy
III. vasodilators, e.g., protacyclin

(A) I and II
(B) I and III
(C) II and III
(D) I, II, and III

76. The chest x-ray with ARDS (adult respiratory distress syndrome) is typically described by which of the following terms?

(A) ground glass
(B) air bronchioles
(C) white-out
(D) bibasilar infiltrates

Questions 77 and 78 refer to the following scenario.

Two days after a lung resection in a 61-year-old, 78-kg male, the physician requests your advice on nutritional replenishment for the patient. He states that, before surgery, he lost

"11 pounds." He is currently receiving 1000 cc of D_5W and 500 cc of NaCl per day. Bowel sounds are present and the patient states that he is hungry. He has the following vital signs:

blood pressure	118/70
pulse	88
respiratory rate	22
temperature	37.8°C

77. Based on the preceding information, how many calories is the patient receiving at the present time?

(A) 170 kcal
(B) 250 kcal
(C) 500 kcal
(D) 1000 kcal

78. Based on the preceding information, which action should be taken?

(A) Start the patient on 1800 cc of a full-strength enteral preparation, e.g., Osmolite or Ensure.
(B) Start the patient on hyperalimentation with 1500 cc of $D_{50}W$ with 10% amino acids.
(C) No action is necessary; the current regime is adequate in meeting nutritional needs.
(D) No enteral feeding should be started, keep the patient on an NPO regime for the first week and increase the D_5W volume to 2000 cc per day.

Questions 79 and 80 refer to the following scenario.

A 56-year-old male is admitted to your unit from the cardiac catheterization laboratory, where an angioplasty of the right coronary artery was performed. He currently has a balloon pump in place, set at an inflation ratio of 1:2. His cardiac output is 5.1, with a blood pressure of 142/82. After admission, he complains of a headache unrelieved by acetaminophen. During the next 24 hours, he is weaned off the balloon pump and it is removed. The headache, however, remains and is unrelieved by acetaminophen plus 30 mg of codeine.

79. Which of the following conditions is possibly developing?

(A) ventricular aneurysm
(B) pericardial tamponade
(C) distal migration of a coronary thrombus into the head
(D) intracerebral bleeding

80. Which of the following actions should be taken?

   I. repeat of the cardiac catheterization
   II. cessation of heparin
   III. administration of thrombolytics

   (A) I
   (B) II
   (C) I and III
   (D) II and III

81. Which component of the immune system has reduced effectiveness in AIDS (acquired immune deficiency syndrome) when the drug cyclosporine is used?

   (A) B lymphocytes
   (B) T4 lymphocytes
   (C) T8 lymphocytes
   (D) neutrophils

82. Pulsus paradoxus is manifested by which of the following symptoms?

   (A) decrease in blood pressure on inspiration
   (B) increase in heart rate on inspiration
   (C) decrease in central venous pressure with the addition of PEEP (positive end expiratory pressure)
   (D) increase in blood pressure on inspiration

Questions 83 and 84 refer to the following scenario.

A 59-year-old female was admitted yesterday to your unit with the diagnosis of sepsis, accompanied by a fever (temperature 39°C). Over the past few hours, she has developed severe shortness of breath and anxiety. Her respiratory rate is 40 bpm and her breathing is labored. Lung sounds are present bilaterally with widespread crackles and scattered wheezes. A chest x ray indicates generalized opacity. Analysis of her blood gases indicates the following:

pH	7.46
$PaCO_2$	30
PaO_2	49
FIO_2	0.60 via face mask

83. Based on the preceding information, which condition is likely to be developing?

(A) severe pneumonia

(B) ARDS (adult respiratory distress syndrome)

(C) generalized atelectasis

(D) cardiogenic pulmonary edema

84. Which of the following treatments would be most appropriate to treat the pulmonary disturbance?

(A) increased oxygen therapy

(B) sedation and diuretics

(C) PEEP (positive end expiratory pressure) or CPAP (continuous positive airway pressure)

(D) bronchodilators

85. Which of the following is responsible for fibrinolytic activity?

(A) plasmin

(B) thrombin

(C) factor I

(D) factor X

86. Which type of treatment would be preferred in reducing excessive bleeding in a patient with hemophilia A?

(A) whole blood

(B) platelets

(C) factor IX

(D) cryoprecipitate

87. A drug that acts to alter spontaneous depolarization of cardiac muscle cells will act in which phase of the action potential?

(A) phase 1

(B) phase 2

(C) phase 3

(D) phase 4

88. A 67-year-old male is admitted to your unit following coronary artery bypass grafting. He is in the unit for 6 hours and is nearly rewarmed to normal body temperature. However, you note that his SvO_2 has fallen from 0.65 to 0.56 during your shift. Which of the following is LEAST likely to be responsible for the fall in the SvO_2 level?

(A) decreased hemoglobin

(B) decreased cardiac output

(C) increased oxygen consumption

(D) decreased PaO_2

89. Treating pancreatic cancer can be surgically attempted by means of which procedure?

    (A) pancreaticoantrectomy
    (B) islet cell transplant
    (C) pancreaticohepatic resection (Lewis procedure)
    (D) pancreatoduodenectomy (Whipple procedure)

Questions 90 and 91 refer to the following scenario.

A 38-year-old female is in the intensive care unit for treatment of hypotension related to sepsis. Her primary diagnosis is metastatic breast cancer. Her current vital signs are listed below:

blood pressure	88/58
pulse	118
respiratory rate	36
temperature	39°C

Earlier in the shift, you noted she had begun spontaneous bleeding from a central IV. The physician ordered coagulation studies, which revealed the following:

platelets	60,000
prothrombin time	30
activated partial thromboplastin time	80
fibrin degradation products	70

90. Based on the preceding information, which condition is likely to be developing?

    (A) von Willebrand's syndrome
    (B) disseminated intravascular clotting
    (C) vitamin K deficiency
    (D) primary platelet dysfunction

91. Which treatment would most likely be given for this condition?

    (A) fresh frozen plasma
    (B) cyroprecipitate
    (C) factor IX
    (D) intravenous vitamin K

92. Mitral valve papillary muscle rupture would initially present with which of the following signs or symptoms?

(A) distended neck veins
(B) systolic murmur
(C) low PCWP (pulmonary capillary wedge pressure)
(D) pulsus paradoxus

93. In a patient with thick airway secretions, which of the following would best aid secretion removal?

    (A) stimulating the cough reflex
    (B) postural drainage
    (C) instillation of saline into the airway
    (D) increasing suction pressure to 300 mm Hg during endotracheal suctioning

94. A patient admitted to your unit after ingestion of a caustic acid solution could be expected to receive which treatment?

    (A) ipecac to induce vomiting
    (B) administration of ammonium chloride
    (C) gastric irrigation with large volumes of water
    (D) immediate exploratory laparotomy

95. Which of the following is/are consistent with symptoms of spinal shock?

    I. loss of autonomic nervous control
    II. loss of sensation below the lesion
    III. flaccid paralysis below the lesion

    (A) I
    (B) I and II
    (C) II and III
    (D) I, II, and III

96. Left ventricular failure alone presents with all of the symptoms listed below but one. Select the symptom that does NOT accompany simple left ventricular failure.

    (A) tachycardia
    (B) increased PCWP (pulmonary capillary wedge pressure)
    (C) increased CVP (central venous pressure)
    (D) shortness of breath

97. Which of the following sets of blood gases values is illustrative of pure respiratory acidosis?

(A) pH 7.28, $PaCO_2$ 22, HCO_3^- 16
(B) pH 7.38, $PaCO_2$ 62, HCO_3^- 36
(C) pH 7.48, $PaCO_2$ 31, HCO_3^- 24
(D) pH 7.22, $PaCO_2$ 62, HCO_3^- 25

98. You are caring for a 37-year-old female admitted with an intracerebral bleed. The nurse on the preceding shift tells you that a neurologic examination was performed on your patient and that she had an abnormal "doll's eyes" test. Which of the following descriptions best describes an abnormal oculocephalic response to the "doll's eyes" test?

(A) Bright light in one eye causes a constriction of the opposite pupil.
(B) The eyes follow the direction of a quick turn of the head.
(C) The eyes tend to remain opposite to the direction of the head turn.
(D) The eyes develop nystagmus following instillation of cold water into the ear.

Questions 99 and 100 refer to the following scenario.

A 25-year-old female is admitted to your unit following a motor vehicle accident. She complains of abdominal pain although no external evidence of trauma exists. Her neurologic examination is normal, although she appears anxious. Vital signs are blood pressure 86/54, pulse 118, respiratory rate 32. She has no specific abdominal pain although left upper quadrant pain is slightly more evident. Bowel sounds are distant but present. Her skin is cool and clammy. As you examine her, you note that her blood pressure falls to 72/48.

99. Based on the preceding information, which condition is likely to be developing?

(A) vasovagal reaction to the accident situation
(B) liver laceration
(C) pancreatic hemorrhage
(D) splenic rupture

100. Which treatment could be expected in this situation?

I. fluid expansion with lactated Ringer's and monitoring of the blood pressure
II. placing a nasogastric tube and performing gastric lavage
III. preparing for an exploratory laparotomy

(A) I and II
(B) I and III
(C) II and III
(D) I, II, and III

101. Interpret the following ECG rhythm strip.

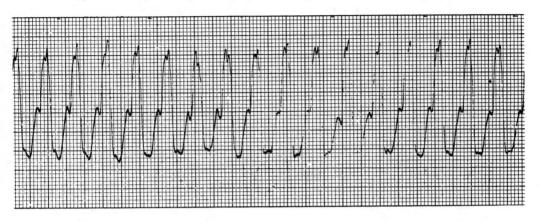

    (A) ventricular tachycardia
    (B) ventricular fibrillation
    (C) atrial tachycardia
    (D) atrial flutter

Questions 102 and 103 refer to the following scenario.

A 55-year-old male is in your unit with the diagnosis of cardiomyopathy. His ejection fraction as measured during a cardiac catheterization is 19%. He is in the unit now with increasing shortness of breath, decreased urine output, and episodes of confusion. His admission ECG indicates ST segment depresssion in leads V_1 to V_4. He currently has a pulmonary artery catheter in place to help in the assessment of his hemodynamics. The following information is available from the catheter:

blood pressure	114/62
pulse	102
CI	2.3
PA	42/26
PCWP	24
CVP	14

102. Based on the preceding information, which situation exists?

    (A) left ventricular failure
    (B) right ventricular failure
    (C) biventricular failure
    (D) anterior wall MI (myocardial infarction)

103. Which therapy is most likely to be effective in improving the ejection fraction in this patient?

(A) dobutamine
(B) oxygen therapy
(C) dopamine
(D) nitroglycerine

104. Nursing care for the immunosuppressed patient includes all of the following EXCEPT:

(A) assessment of the mouth and throat
(B) taking only rectal temperatures
(C) avoiding live flowers and plants in the room
(D) enteral as opposed to parenteral nutrition

105. Which of the following statements best describe the high mortality associated with the person who progresses from sepsis to septic shock?

I. Antibiotic therapy is NOT effective in controlling the septic response.
II. The release of myocardial depressant factors limits cardiac compensatory mechanisms.
III. Immune system suppression occurs from the septic cascade.

(A) I and II
(B) I and III
(C) II and III
(D) I, II, and III

106. An inferior MI (myocardial infarction) is manifested on the 12-lead ECG in which of the following leads?

(A) V_1 to V_4
(B) I, aVL, V_5, V_6
(C) V_{3R} to V_{6R}
(D) II, III, and aVF

107. Which of the following is NOT an appropriate parameter to measure to determine adequacy for weaning from mechanical ventilation?

(A) minute ventilation
(B) tidal volume
(C) peak inspiratory pressure
(D) forced expiratory volume in one second (FEV_1)

Questions 108 and 109 refer to the following scenario.

A 65-year-old male is admitted to your unit following a coronary artery bypass graft and valve replacement. During your shift, he complains of left-side chest pain. His lung sounds are clear, he does not complain of shortness of breath, and he has an SpO_2 value of 0.92 on 40% oxygen. His mediastinal chest tube has drained 10 cc on your shift. His hemodynamics are listed below.

blood pressure	112/70
pulse	112
CI	2.0
PA	32/20
PCWP	19
CVP	19

108. Based on the preceding information, which condition is likely to be developing?

    (A) left ventricular failure
    (B) right ventricular failure
    (C) pericardial tamponade
    (D) pulmonary emboli

109. What would be the most appropriate therapy to treat this situation?

    (A) dobutamine
    (B) stripping of the mediastinal tube
    (C) thrombolytics
    (D) pericardiocentesis

Questions 110 and 111 refer to the following scenario.

A 31-year-old male is admitted to your unit with ARD (acute respiratory distress). He has lost weight over the past few weeks, has a generalized lymphadenopathy, and is febrile (39.5°C). He has been told in the past his blood tested positive for the HIV (human immunodeficiency virus).

110. Based on the preceding information, what is the most likely cause of the ARD?

    (A) *Pneumocystis carinii* pneumonia
    (B) *Hemophilus influenzae* pneumonia
    (C) ARDS (adult respiratory distress syndrome)
    (D) Kaposi's sarcoma

111. Aside from oxygenation and ventilation support, treatment for this condition would most likely include which therapy?

(A) aminoglycosides
(B) ticarcillin
(C) pentamidine
(D) amphotericin

112. Right ventricular infarctions are best seen in which of the following leads?

(A) V_1 to V_4
(B) I, aVL, V_5, V_6
(C) V_{3R} to V_{6R}
(D) II, III, and aVF

113. A 31-year-old female is admitted to your unit following a motor vehicle accident in which she received crush injuries to the chest. She currently is intubated and on AMV (assist/control mechanical ventilation). Her PaO_2 is not responding to oxygen therapy so the physician decides to add PEEP (positive end expiratory pressure) to her therapy. In monitoring the effectiveness of the PEEP, which parameters should be present to indicate an appropriate response to the therapy?

I. maintenance of cardiac output
II. increase in PaO_2 and SaO_2
III. reduced pulmonary compliance

(A) I and II
(B) I and III
(C) II and III
(D) I, II, and III

Questions 114 and 115 refer to the following scenario.

A 24-year-old female is admitted in an unresponsive condition to your unit. No overt signs of trauma are present. Vital signs include blood pressure 110/80, pulse 96, respiratory rate 21, and temperature 37.5°C. Shortly after admission to the unit, she has a generalized seizure. A subsequent head CT (computed tomographic) scan is negative and a neurologic examination reveals no abnormalities. Laboratory serum data indicate the following:

Na^+	111
K^+	3.3
Cl^-	74
HCO_3^-	25
PaO_2	61
$PaCO_2$	34
pH	7.43

114. Based on the preceding information, which condition is likely to be the cause of the neurologic symptoms?

(A) hypoxemia
(B) pontomedullary hemorrhage
(C) hypokalemia
(D) hyponatremia

115. Correction of the abnormal sodium should be done slowly in order to avoid which of the following?

   I. fluid overload
  II. cerebral injury
 III. exacerbation of hypoxemia

    (A) I
    (B) I and III
    (C) II
    (D) I, II, and III

116. Which of the following is an indication of an aberrantly conducted APC (atrial premature contraction) versus a PVC (premature ventricular contraction)?

(A) rsR′ in V_1
(B) precordial concordancy
(C) Rr′ in V_1
(D) extreme right axis deviation

117. Which of the following is the best indicator of alveolar ventilation?

(A) PaO_2 levels
(B) minute ventilation
(C) $PaCO_2$ values
(D) respiratory rate

Questions 118 and 119 refer to the following scenario.

A 71-year-old female returns to your unit from the cardiac catheterization laboratory. While in the cath lab, she was noted to have 70% obstruction of her left anterior descending artery, 95% obstruction of her circumflex artery, and 60% obstruction of her right coronary artery. An angioplasty was performed on her circumflex artery, which reduced the degree of obstruction to 30%.

118. If she was to develop a reocclusion of the circumflex artery, which type of MI (myocardial infarction) could occur?

(A) anterior
(B) inferior
(C) lateral
(D) posterior

119. Which type of reperfusion dysrhythmias are likely to occur in the first 24 hours postangioplasty?

I. ventricular ectopy (PVCs; premature ventricular contractions)
II. bundle branch blocks
III. bradycardias

(A) I and II
(B) I and III
(C) II and III
(D) I, II, and III

Questions 120 and 121 refer to the following scenario.

Following a subtotal thyroidectomy, your patient develops an increased heart rate (120) and temperature (39.7°C). She becomes confused, disoriented, and agitated. Her blood pressure changes from 130/78 to 170/100. Breath sounds are equal, and a neurologic examination is normal except for the presence of agitation and confusion. Analysis of her blood gases reveal the following:

pH	7.47
$PaCO_2$	32
PaO_2	90
FIO_2	room air

120. Based on the preceding information, which condition would you suspect is most likely to be developing?

(A) parathyroid storm
(B) cerebral hemorrhage
(C) pulmonary emboli
(D) thyroid storm

121. Which initial treatment would most likely be administered?

(A) calcium gluconate
(B) heparin
(C) Inderal (propranolol)
(D) thyroxine

122. A 22-year-old female is admitted to your unit for treatment of a supraventricular tachycardia. Which of the following medications may be employed to try to terminate this dysrhythmia?

   I. Verapamil
  II. adenosine
 III. esmolol

    (A) I and II
    (B) I and III
    (C) II and III
    (D) I, II, and III

123. PSV (pressure support ventilation) differs from IMV (intermittent mandatory ventilation) and AMV (assist/control mechanical ventilation) in which of the following ways?

    (A) Volumes are delivered within pressure limits.
    (B) Volumes are delivered within time limits.
    (C) PSV is useful when the pulmonary compliance is at least 15 cm H_2O, whereas IMV and AMV can only be used at 10 cm H_2O.
    (D) PSV requires a preset tidal volume.

124. A 39-year-old male is in your unit after being found in an unresponsive state in the city park. He currently responds to deep, painful stimuli. He has no identification and no past medical history, although his clothes have the odor of alcohol. His vital signs and laboratory data are as follows:

blood pressure	116/68
pulse	96
respiratory rate	29
temperature	36.6°C
Na^+	135
K^+	3.9
Cl^-	100
HCO_3^-	22
BUN	92
glucose	196
SGOT	652
alkaline phosphatase	155
lactate	14

Based on the preceding information, which condition is likely to be present?

    (A) hepatic encephalopathy
    (B) diabetic coma
    (C) hepatorenal syndrome
    (D) portacaval syndrome

125. A 43-year-old male is admitted to your unit following a motorcycle accident. He was thrown from the cycle and skidded 150 feet in gravel along the side of the road. He now has multiple contusions and abrasions, although his neurologic examination is unremarkable. He does, however, develop a rhabdomyolysis with a resultant lactic acidosis. His current laboratory data are as follows:

pH	7.28
PaO_2	81
$PaCO_2$	33
HCO_3^-	19
lactate	4
Na^+	138
K^+	5.4
Cl^-	104

In this situation, the house officer wants to treat the potassium level of 5.4. What is the relationship between potassium and the lactic acidosis seen in this situation?

(A) as pH increases, K^+ decreases
(B) as pH decreases, K^+ increases
(C) as pH decreases, K^+ decreases
(D) as pH increases, K^+ increases

126. Unstable angina is differentiated from stable angina by which of the following?

(A) chest pain at rest
(B) Q wave development on the ECG
(C) ST segment depression in affected leads
(D) chest pain relieved by nitroglycerine

Questions 127 and 128 refer to the following scenario.

A 52-year-old male with the diagnosis of lymphocytic leukemia is admitted to your unit with mild hypotension, hypoxemia, and shortness of breath. He is placed on AMV (assist/control mechanical ventilation), tidal volume (VT) 750 cc, respiratory rate 12, total rate 33, FIO_2 0.70. He is very anxious and requires sedation to alleviate the anxiety. A pulmonary artery catheter is inserted and blood gases drawn. The following information is obtained:

blood pressure	108/66
pulse	116
CO	4
CI	2.3
PA	46/30

PCWP	10
CVP	10
PaO_2	56
$PaCO_2$	32
pH	7.36
HCO_3^-	23

127. Based on the preceding information, which condition is developing?

(A) noncardiogenic pulmonary edema
(B) cardiogenic pulmonary edema
(C) right ventricular failure causing pulmonary edema
(D) hypovolemia

128. Which strategy would be followed in the treatment of this patient?

(A) Administer fluids to increase the PCWP (pulmonary capillary wedge pressure).
(B) Give diuretics to keep the PCWP as low as possible.
(C) Give bicarbonate to treat the metabolic acidosis.
(D) Administer dopamine to support the failing left ventricle.

129. What is the cerebral perfusion pressure in a patient with the following information?

blood pressure	100/70
ICP	15
CVP	10
PCWP	8

(A) 40
(B) 55
(C) 60
(D) 65

130. A 46-year-old male is admitted to your unit with the diagnosis of an epidural hematoma following a motor vehicle accident. Which artery is usually involved when a head injury produces an epidural bleed?

(A) internal carotid
(B) middle meningeal
(C) anterior communicating
(D) parietal

131. For what does the first letter in DVI [pacemaker] stand?

(A) digital signal processing
(B) dual chamber sensing mechanisms
(C) dual chamber pacing
(D) diverse programmability features

132. A 30-year-old female is admitted to your unit with the diagnosis of possible pulmonary emboli. The following information is available to aid in the diagnosis:

pH	7.36
$PaCO_2$	32
PaO_2	77
HCO_3-	23
dead space (VT)	45%
End tidal CO_2 ($PETCO_2$)	20

Based on the preceding information, are enough data present to establish the diagnosis of pulmonary embolism?

(A) Yes, dead space measurements are definitive for pulmonary embolism.
(B) Yes, the $PaCO_2$-$PETCO_2$ gradient confirms a pulmonary embolism.
(C) No, a ventilation perfusion scan is needed.
(D) No, pulmonary angiography is the optimal method to confirm a pulmonary embolism.

133. Aldosterone production is stimulated by which event?

(A) renin-angiotension release
(B) systemic hypertension
(C) hypernatremia
(D) parathyroid release

Questions 134 and 135 refer to the following scenario.

A 27-year-old female presents to the intensive care unit with hypotension and respiratory distress following initial chemotherapy for acute myelogenous leukemia. A pulmonary artery catheter is placed to help manage the hemodynamics. Vital signs and laboratory data are as follows:

blood pressure	94/62
pulse	113
respiratory rate	32
temperature	40°C

CI	6.2
PA	27/11
PCWP	9
CVP	3
PaO_2	68
$PaCO_2$	34
pH	7.36
FIO_2	0.80
platelets	21,000
white blood cells	900
segmented neutrophils	30%
banded neutrophils	20%
lymphocytes	35%

134. Based on the preceding information, which condition is likely to be developing?

(A) ARDS (adult respiratory distress syndrome)
(B) CHF (congestive heart failure)
(C) graft-versus-host reaction
(D) systemic inflammatory response syndrome

135. Which nursing or medical intervention would NOT be necessary based on the preceding information?

(A) reverse isolation
(B) bleeding precautions
(C) administration of triple antibiotic coverage
(D) intubation

136. During your shift, a 79-year-old male who has been admitted for CHF (congestive heart failure) develops a bradycardia (ventricular escape rhythm). He becomes hypotensive and his level of consciousness decreases. Which of the following is a reason why a transcutaneous pacemaker would be preferable to a transvenous pacemaker under this circumstance?

(A) better capture ability
(B) less painful
(C) easier to apply
(D) smaller-sized equipment

137. Cardiac contusion is best identified by which of the following techniques?

(A) creatine phosphokinase (CPK) MB isoenzyme analysis
(B) ECG change analysis
(C) chest x ray
(D) echocardiography

138. Physical assessment of the abdomen should take place in which sequence?

(A) inspection, deep palpation, light palpation, percussion
(B) deep palpation, light palpation, percussion, inspection
(C) light palpation, inspection, deep palpation, percussion
(D) inspection, light palpation, percussion, deep palpation

139. Which test measures the presence of an antibody (to ABO antigens) on a red blood cell?

(A) Coombs's test
(B) indirect Coombs's test
(C) complement fixation studies
(D) histamine fixation

140. A patient with a C-6 fracture would most likely be able to perform which of the following movements?

(A) no movements of any kind
(B) movement from the waist up
(C) movement of only the shoulders and fingers
(D) some crude walking movements

141. A 62-year-old male is admitted to your unit with a diagnosis of non–Q wave MI (myocardial infarction). He was transferred from another hospital, where he was admitted initially two days ago. In order to confirm the diagnosis of MI, which test would most likely be performed?

(A) creatine phosphokinase (CPK) MB isoenzyme analysis
(B) ECG
(C) echocardiogram
(D) lactic acid dehydrogenase (LDH) isoenzyme analysis

142. A 27-year-old female is in your unit following a single right lung transplant. On your shift, she complains of shortness of breath. Upon auscultation, you hear diminished breath sounds on the right. You are able to palpate crepitations (subcutaneous emphysema) in her neck and upper chest. Her pulse oximeter is reading 0.93, down from 0.99. Based on this information, which condition is likely to be developing?

(A) pulmonary emboli
(B) pleural rupture and hemothorax
(C) bronchial tear
(D) pneumopericardium

143. In the following ECG rhythm strip, identify any abnormality which is present.

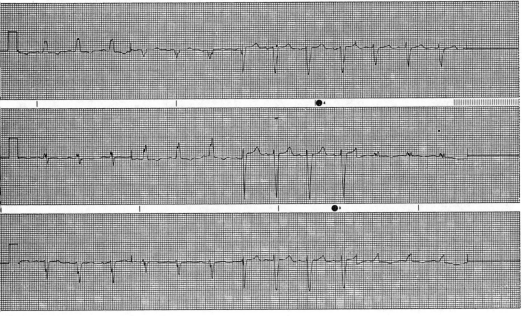

    (A) left bundle branch block
    (B) anterior hemiblock
    (C) right bundle branch block
    (D) posterior hemiblock

144. An upper motor neuron lesion presents with which of the following symptoms?

    (A) hypertension and bradycardia
    (B) muscle flaccidity
    (C) muscle spasticity
    (D) cognitive defects

145. Which antibody mediates hypersensitivity (allergic) reactions?

    (A) IgG
    (B) IgM
    (C) IgA
    (D) IgE

Questions 146 and 147 refer to the following scenario.

A 65-year-old female is admitted to your unit in an unresponsive state, with blood pressure 80/48, pulse 122, and skin that is cool and clammy to the touch. Her family states that she was healthy until after supper that evening, when she suddenly slumped over in her chair. A central line is inserted along with a pulmonary artery catheter. The catheter reveals the following information:

PA	42/25
PCWP	24
CVP	16
CO	3.4
CI	1.6

146. Based on the preceding information, which condition is likely to be developing?

    (A) hypovolemic shock
    (B) pericardial tamponade
    (C) sepsis
    (D) cardiogenic shock

147. Which medication would most effectively raise her blood pressure at this time?

    (A) dopamine
    (B) dobutamine
    (C) nitroprusside
    (D) Lasix

148. Following a code for a cardiopulmonary arrest on an 83-year-old male, the physician suspects that a flail chest injury may be present secondary to aggressive CPR (cardiopulmonary resuscitation). If flail chest is present, which of the following would be seen?

    (A) paradoxical movement of portions of the chest with inspiration
    (B) expansion of both the chest and the abdomen on inspiration
    (C) outward expansion of at least two locations of the chest wall during expiration
    (D) a cracking sound in the chest during breathing

149. An ICP (intracranial pressure) tracing with the presence of A waves at a pressure of 10 mm Hg indicates which of the following?

(A) cerebral hypoxia
(B) increasing ICP
(C) impending seizures
(D) normal ICP

150. A 61-year-old female is in your unit with the diagnosis of CHF (congestive heart failure). She develops a series of dysrhythmias, which include aberrantly conducted APCs (atrial premature contractions) with both left and right bundle branch block characteristics. Which lead is most likely to detect the left and right bundle branch block characteristics?

(A) lead avL
(B) lead II
(C) MCL_1 lead
(D) MCL_3 lead

151. Which category of drugs is most helpful in relieving unstable angina?

(A) preload reducers
(B) beta blockers
(C) parasympathetic inhibitors
(D) contractility agents

Questions 152 and 153 refer to the following scenario.

A 71-year-old female is in her fourth day in the intensive care unit with left lower lobe pneumonia. Her present antibiotic regime includes gentamycin and imipenem. She is currently intubated and receiving mechanical ventilation with the following settings:

mode	IMV
V_T	750 cc
respiratory rate	12
total rate	27
FIO_2	0.60

Her blood pressure is stable at 128/84, and her urine output has been 750 cc over the past 24 hours. Her current laboratory data reveal the following information:

PaO_2	71
$PaCO_2$	44
pH	7.35
creatinine	2.4
BUN	40

152. Based on the preceding information, which type of organisms is the antibiotic therapy attempting to affect?

(A) pulmonary gram-positive bacteria
(B) pulmonary gram-negative bacteria
(C) systemic fungi
(D) systemic viruses

153. Which treatment is most likely to improve the intrapulmonary shunt in this situation?

(A) addition of PEEP (positive end expiratory pressure)
(B) normal saline bolus
(C) changing antibiotics
(D) diuretics

154. A 36-year-old male is in your unit with a diagnosis of cardiomyopathy. He is currently unresponsive to dobutamine therapy. Which other inotrope might be employed to improve his hemodynamics?

(A) epinephrine
(B) phenylephrine
(C) digoxin
(D) amrinone

155. Which of the following medications would be most likely to stimulate gastrointestinal motility?

(A) atropine
(B) epinephrine
(C) edrophonium (Tensilon)
(D) dopamine

156. Which of the following interventions is most appropriate for pain relief due to unstable angina?

(A) angioplasty
(B) IABP (intraaortic balloon pump) use
(C) CABG (coronary artery bypass grafting)
(D) cardiac transplantation

Questions 157 and 158 refer to the following scenario.

A 65-year-old female is in your unit following surgery to repair a ruptured small intestine. She has been in the unit for five days and has developed respiratory distress requiring mechanical ventilation. She is currently arousable upon stimulation and is confused, but has no complaints other than incisional discomfort. She has the following vital signs and laboratory information:

blood pressure	94/58
pulse	114
respiratory rate	28
temperature	38.9°C
pH	7.33
PaO_2	77
$PaCO_2$	36
HCO_3^-	20
FIO_2	0.60
LDH	496
SGOT	517
white blood cells	23,000

157. Based on the preceding information, which condition is likely to be developing?

    (A) multisystem organ failure
    (B) renal failure
    (C) hepatic failure
    (D) meningeal irritation

158. Which of the following therapies is considered curative for this situation?

    (A) antibiotic therapy
    (B) mechanical ventilation and oxygenation support
    (C) administration of osmotic diuretics
    (D) No therapies are curative for this situation.

159. Hepatic encephalopathy is frequently preceded by which physical symptom?

    (A) Trousseau's sign
    (B) asterixis
    (C) positive Babinski (extensor plantar) reflex
    (D) Warner's sign

160. A 51-year-old male is admitted to your unit with shortness of breath, crackles scattered throughout both lung fields, 3+ pitting edema of the lower extremities, and an SpO_2 (pulse oximeter) value of 0.88. The following hemodynamic information is available:

CI	2.6
PA	51/34
PCWP	13
CVP	19

Based on the preceding information, which condition is likely to be developing?

(A) left ventricular failure
(B) biventricular failure
(C) right ventricular failure
(D) ARDS (adult respiratory distress syndrome)

161. Thrombolytic therapy for MI (myocardial infarction) should be undertaken when which of the following criteria has been met?

(A) Q wave formation to document presence of MI
(B) ST segment depression in consecutive leads
(C) pain should be relieved by nitroglycerine
(D) pain should be less than four hours old

162. A 32-year-old male is in your unit after sustaining a blunt trauma to the head. His pupillary response changes from one in which the pupils are bilaterally equal and responsive to one in which the left pupil is responsive but the right pupil is unresponsive to light and dilated. What does this pattern of responses indicate?

(A) central herniation
(B) uncal herniation
(C) anterior cord compression
(D) optic nerve compression

Questions 163 and 164 refer to the following scenario.

A 27-year-old female is admitted to your unit with the diagnosis of acute exacerbation of asthma. Wheezing is prominent thoughout both lungs. Breath sounds are equal and easily heard. Blood gas analysis and vital signs indicate the following:

PaO_2	76
$PaCO_2$	32
pH	7.44
blood pressure	134/76
pulse	110
respiratory rate	30

Shortly after admission, she complains of increasing shortness of breath. Listening to her lungs, you note that the wheezing and breath sounds have decreased. Blood gas values and vital signs are now as follows:

PaO_2	70
$PaCO_2$	43
pH	7.35

blood pressure	150/88
pulse	120
respiratory rate	38

163. Based on the preceding information, which condition is likely to be developing?

    (A) pneumothorax secondary to increased mean airway pressures with auto-PEEP (positive end expiratory pressure) from the asthma
    (B) pulmonary emboli
    (C) worsening alveolar airflow
    (D) right heart failure complicating the asthma situation

164. Which treatment would be least effective at this time?

    (A) subcutaneous epinephrine
    (B) aerosolized beta stimulants
    (C) intravenous theophylline
    (D) intravenous atropine

165. A 34-year-old fireman is admitted to your unit following smoke inhalation injury. He states he was entering a room when a "ball of fire" exploded in front of him. During which time period would he be at greatest risk for developing pulmonary edema from the inhalation injury?

    (A) during the first 2 hours
    (B) 4 to 12 hours
    (C) 12 to 24 hours
    (D) >24 hours

166. IABP (intraaortic balloon pump) therapy produces two direct physiologic benefits. Identify these two benefits from the choices below.

    (A) decreases preload and afterload
    (B) increases coronary perfusion and decreases afterload
    (C) increases coronary perfusion and decreases preload
    (D) increases contractility and preload

167. Following a femoral-iliac arterial resection, which positions are appropriate during the immediate postoperative period?

    I. semi-Fowler's
    II. supine
    III. left lateral

        (A) I and II
        (B) I and III
        (C) II and III
        (D) I, II, and III

168. Based on the hypoxemic drive to breath concept, which of the following patients would be most at risk for developing respiratory depression with the administration of excessive oxygen therapy?

(A) chronic bronchitic patient with pH 7.34, PaO_2 56, $PaCO_2$ 68
(B) emphysematous patient with pH 7.37, PaO_2 56, $PaCO_2$ 35
(C) asthmatic patient with pH 7.24, PaO_2 79, $PaCO_2$ 58
(D) COPD (chronic obstructive pulmonary disease) patient with pH 7.44, PaO_2 64, $PaCO_2$ 39

Questions 169 and 170 refer to the following scenario.

A 57-year-old male is admitted to your unit for investigation of the cause of an acute onset of abdominal pain. He has a history of alcohol abuse. He states that he has had abdominal pain for several days but that the pain became acutely worse today. Currently he states that he is in severe epigastric pain with radiation to the back. The abdomen is tender but no guarding is exhibited. Chvostek's and Trousseau's signs are present. Serum amylase is elevated.

169. Based on the preceding information, which condition is likely to be developing?

(A) acute pancreatitis
(B) bowel obstruction
(C) superior mesenteric artery occlusion
(D) abdominal aortic aneurysm

170. Which treatment would most likely be avoided in this condition?

(A) placing the patient on an NPO (non per os; nothing by mouth) regimen
(B) starting nasogastric suction
(C) pain relief with meperidine (Demerol)
(D) surgery to remove the causative pancreatic area

171. The simultaneous use of nitroprusside and dobutamine is intended to work through which of the following actions?

(A) decrease preload and increase afterload
(B) increase contractility through reducing preload
(C) decrease SVR (systemic vascular resistance) and improve contractility
(D) increase cerebral perfusion pressure and baroreceptor stimulation

172. A 57-year-old female has been in your unit for two weeks and is diagnosed as having multisystem organ failure. (MSOF). On the 15th day she develops a fever that reaches 41°C. Which condition is likely to be developing?

(A) inflammatory response to multisystem organ failure
(B) failure of central thermoregulation
(C) probable viral infection and infectious response
(D) bacterial inflammatory response

173. Which of the following is NOT a strong afterload-reducing agent?

(A) nicardipine
(B) labetalol
(C) nitroprusside
(D) nitroglycerine

Questions 174 and 175 refer to the following scenario.

Following head trauma from a hammer blow, a 45-year-old male is admitted to your unit after evacuation of a subdural hematoma. Initial postoperative neurologic checks reveal equally responsive pupils and appropriate limb movement. During your shift he begins to complain of headache and nausea. He is confused as to time and place. His respiratory rate increases to 24 from 18.

174. Which of the preceding signs is not an indication of increasing ICP (intracranial pressure)?

(A) nausea
(B) headache
(C) increased respiratory rate
(D) development of confusion

175. Which of the following nursing measures would help reduce the ICP (intracranial pressure)?

(A) keeping the head in a neutral position
(B) turning the head to the right to aid choroid plexus absorption of CSF (cerebrospinal fluid)
(C) increasing the frequency of suctioning while administering 100% oxygen
(D) adding PEEP (positive end expiratory pressure) to reduce inflow of blood to the brain

Questions 176 and 177 refer to the following scenario.

A 71-year-old male is admitted to your unit with increasing shortness of breath. He has a history of COPD (chronic obstructive pulmonary disease). His current medications are Lasix (furosemide) (40 mg daily), potassium (40 mEq daily), and Theo-Dur (theophylline) (300 mg daily). He has dependent edema and distended neck veins. Crackles are heard thoughout both lung fields. Analysis of his blood gases on admission reveals the following:

PaO$_2$	59
PaCO$_2$	54
pH	7.33
FIO$_2$	0.30

During your shift, he becomes hypotensive and a pulmonary artery catheter is placed. The catheter reveals the following:

CI	2.2
PA	66/38
PCWP	13
CVP	20

176. Based on the preceding information, which condition is present?

(A) cardiac tamponade
(B) secondary active pulmonary hypertension
(C) ARDS (adult respiratory distress syndrome)
(D) biventricular failure

177. Which treatment would be most effective in reducing the pulmonary arterial pressure?

I. oxygen therapy
II. aminophylline
III. Lasix

(A) I and II
(B) I and III
(C) II and III
(D) I, II, and III

178. When listening to a patient's lungs, you note that crackles are present throughout both lungs. The patient is not orthopneic and the lung sounds do not change with position. He has "swelling of the feet and hands." Distended jugular veins are present. Which of the following conditions could be present based on this information?

I. pulmonary disease (right ventricular failure)
II. cardiac disease (left ventricular failure)
III. biventricular failure

(A) I only
(B) I and III
(C) II only
(D) I, II, and III

179. A patient admitted with hyperparathyroidism would most likely benefit from which of the following treatments?

(A) thyroxine
(B) vitamin K
(C) fluid bolus with normal saline
(D) calcium gluconate

180. You are caring for a 78-year-old female with exacerbation of CHF (congestive heart failure). The following data are available for assessment:

blood pressure	124/74
CO	3.6
CI	1.8
PCWP	16
CVP	12
SV	33
SI	16
EF	31%

Give an example of therapies that would be most effective in treating these hemodynamics.

   I. dobutamine
  II. captopril
 III. Lasix
   (A) I and II
   (B) I and III
   (C) II and III
   (D) I, II, and III

181. A 61-year-old female develops ventricular fibrillation while you are watching the monitor. What is the sequence of actions you should take to reestablish stable hemodynamics in this situation? (Assume you have established pulselessness.)

   I. defibrillate initially at 200 joules
  II. defibrillate at least three times if pulse does not return
 III. start a dopamine drip to increase blood pressure
   (A) I and II
   (B) I and III
   (C) II and III
   (D) I, II, and III

182. In the same patient, you note the following electrolyte values on the first postoperative day:

serum Na^+	111
serum osmolality	272
urine Na^+	32
urine osmolality	322

Based on these values, which treatment would most likely be instituted?

(A) normal saline bolus
(B) fluid restriction or diuretics
(C) increase free water intravenous rate (D_5W)
(D) hyperventilation

Questions 183 and 184 refer to the following scenario.

A 48-year-old male is admitted to your unit following a cardiopulmonary arrest. He was admitted two days ago for investigation of a cerebral mass. He is currently being ventilated at an AMV (assist/control mechanical ventilation) rate of 12, with 10 spontaneous breaths in addition to the ventilator rate. Vital signs include blood pressure 142/86, pulse 104, temperature 37.1°C. Laboratory data reveal the following:

PaO_2	91
$PaCO_2$	32
pH	7.26
Na^+	141
K^+	4.9
Cl^-	101
HCO_3^-	17
glucose	54 mg/dL
oxygen transport	465 cc
creatinine	5
BUN	60

183. Based on the preceding information, which condition is present?

(A) non–anion gap acidosis
(B) hyperkalemia-induced metabolic alkalosis
(C) compensated metabolic alkalosis
(D) anion gap acidosis

184. Which therapies would be employed to help improve the level of consciousness in this patient?

I. increase oxygen delivery
II. increase glucose
III. increase HCO_3^-

(A) I and II
(B) I and III
(C) II and III
(D) I, II, and III

185. A 73-year-old male is transferred to your unit following a hypotensive episode on the floor. His original diagnosis is sepsis secondary to an above-the-knee amputation. The following laboratory data are available:

Na$^+$	142
K$^+$	4.1
Cl$^-$	103
HCO$_3^-$	17
glucose	123
BUN	38
lactate	15
pH	7.29
PaO$_2$	66
PaCO$_2$	29
FIO$_2$	0.50

Based on the preceding information, the physician believes this patient to have cellular hypoxia. Which of the conditions listed are consistent with this diagnosis?

  I. increased intrapulmonary shunt (a/A ratio is 0.21)
 II. lactate of 15
III. pH of 7.29

   (A) I and II
   (B) I and III
   (C) II and III
   (D) I, II, and III

186. A 51-year-old male with chronic atrial fibrillation is admitted to your unit. Which of the following therapies may be employed to treat this condition?

  I. cardioversion at 200 Joules
 II. surgical resection of accessory pathways
III. digoxin

   (A) I and II
   (B) I and III
   (C) II and III
   (D) I, II, and III

Questions 187 and 188 refer to the following scenario.

Following blunt trauma to the head, a 17-year-old male is admitted to your unit for observation. He is alert and oriented although anxious to leave. Over the next hour, you notice that he has ecchymotic development around both eyes. His level of consciousness is unchanged.

187. What is a common name for the above clinical picture?

   (A) Battle's sign
   (B) Homan's sign
   (C) raccoon eyes
   (D) mask eyes

188. Based on the preceding information, which condition may be developing?

(A) temporal skull fracture involving falx cerebri
(B) uncal herniation
(C) fracture of both eye orbits
(D) basilar skull fracture in the anterior fossa

189. A 54-year-old, obese male is admitted to your unit two days after right femoral-popliteal bypass surgery with a complaint of shortness of breath. Upon examination, you note that he is very anxious and appears dyspneic, although the difficulty in breathing is unaffected by position changes. Pulses in the legs are good, although the right leg is more edematous than the left. The right leg feels warmer to the touch than the left. His body temperature is 38.5°C. Analysis of his blood gases reveals the following:

PaO_2	63
$PaCO_2$	34
pH	7.46

Based on the preceding data, which condition is likely to be causing the shortness of breath?

(A) pulmonary emboli
(B) CHF (congestive heart failure)
(C) pneumonia
(D) initial stages of ARDS (adult respiratory distress syndrome)

190. Which nursing measure would most likely improve his shortness of breath?

(A) place him in an upright position
(B) increase the frequency of deep breathing and coughing
(C) sedate him with morphine
(D) perform oral or nasal suctioning at routine intervals

191. Which of the following are potential improved therapies in the treatment of sepsis?

I. interleukin 2
II. steroids
III. monoclonol antibodies

(A) I and II
(B) I and III
(C) II and III
(D) I, II, and III

192. A 69-year-old male is in your unit with a diagnosis of CHF (congestive heart failure). Dobutamine is started at 0800 in an attempt to improve his hemodynamics. From the following information, was the addition of dobutamine helpful?

	0400	0800	1200
blood pressure	108/72	90/62	94/66
pulse	112	92	102
CI	2.1	2.1	2.2
PCWP	18	24	19
CVP	11	13	10
SV	36	39	38

(A) yes, based on the increased CI
(B) yes, based on the decreased PCWP
(C) no, based on increased heart rate
(D) no, based on the absence of improvement in SV

193. A 21-year-old male is admitted following a motor vehicle accident in which he was thrown from the car. At the scene, he had a Glasgow Coma Score of 7. Currently he opens his eyes to painful stimuli, manifests unintelligible verbal responses, and has decorticate posturing (abnormal flexion). Based on his current responses, what is the present Glasgow Coma Score?

(A) 3
(B) 7
(C) 10
(D) 15

194. Beta cells in the pancreas are responsible for producing which of the following substances?

(A) insulin
(B) glucagon
(C) trypsin
(D) plasminogen

195. A 44-year-old male is in your unit following surgery for hepatic resection. During the fourth postoperative day, he develops a temperature of 39°C. His vital signs are as follows:

blood pressure	100/64
pulse	120
respiratory rate	32

Which of the following would be considered accurate statements regarding the elevation in the temperature?

    I. The temperature accounts for the heart rate change.
    II. The temperature is protective rather than harmful.
    III. The increased respiratory rate reflects an increased metabolic rate.

    (A) I and II
    (B) I and III
    (C) II and III
    (D) I, II, and III

Questions 196 and 197 refer to the following scenario.

A 43-year-old secretary is directly admitted to your unit from her physician's office for evaluation of a recent onset of extremity paralysis. Her husband brought her to the physician when she could not move this morning. She had been feeling better after an episode of measles over a week ago but started feeling weak yesterday and today could not move. Examination reveals sensation and tingling in the legs and arms but no movement. She noticed that the symptoms started in her hands and feet and moved up her arms and legs.

196. Based on the preceding information, which condition is likely to be developing?

    (A) Guillain-Barré syndrome
    (B) myasthenia gravis
    (C) amyotrophic lateral sclerosis
    (D) multiple sclerosis

197. Which nursing measure should be taken at least daily to assess the adequacy of her ability to take a deep breath and maintain spontaneous breathing?

    (A) FEV_1 (forced expiratory volume in one second)
    (B) vital capacity
    (C) dynamic compliance
    (D) oxygen gas diffusion testing

198. Intubation of the trachea has several potential complications. Which of the following is NOT a likely complication of attempting tracheal intubation?

    (A) vocal cord injury
    (B) right mainstem intubation
    (C) left mainstem intubation
    (D) esophageal intubation

199. Which of the following parameters is NOT effectively treated by continuous arteriovenous hemofiltration?

(A) creatinine
(B) serum volume
(C) potassium
(D) albumin

200. A cardiologist requests that you maintain the PCWP (pulmonary capillary wedge pressure) at 20 mm Hg, based on the patient's history of CHF (congestive heart failure). From the data given below, is this request valid?

	1600	1800	2000	2200
blood pressure	102/70	92/64	98/68	104/70
pulse	104	90	102	92
CI	1.9	2.1	2.1	2.4
PA	44/25	32/18	39/24	49/26
PCWP	24	16	22	25
CVP	13	8	11	14
SI	18	23	21	24

(A) yes, based on the increased SI over time
(B) yes, based on the increased blood pressure over time
(C) no, since the PA pressures have not stabilized
(D) no, since the PCWP near 20 does not have optimal SI

CONGRATULATIONS!

You have finished the exam. Review it to cover any problematic questions. Do not change any answers unless you are sure the change is necessary. Compare your results with the answers beginning on p. 346. Do not immediately grade your test. After reviewing the exam, take some time to relax before returning to grade your test and study any areas you missed. Note the areas in which you need improvement. This test is an approximation of the actual CCRN exam and should give you a rough idea of how you will do on the exam. Reread in the text any areas in which your success rate was less than 70%. We wish you luck in the actual exam. You are to be congratulated for taking the time and effort to prepare for it.

CHAPTER 10

Comprehensive Practice Exam—2

Questions 1 and 2 refer to the following scenario.

A 76-year-old male is admitted to your unit with the diagnosis of acute inferior wall MI (myocardial infarction). He has a history of COPD (chronic obstructive pulmonary disease) as well. During your shift he begins to complain of shortness of breath. He has crackles one-third of the way up his posterior lobes along with expiratory wheezing. He has an S_3 (gallop) and a II/VI systolic murmur. The following hemodynamic information is available:

blood pressure	100/58
pulse	112
CI	2.1
CO	4.6
PA	38/23
PCWP	21
CVP	13

1. Based on the preceding information, what is likely to be happening?

    (A) exacerbation of the COPD
    (B) development of right ventricular failure
    (C) development of right and left ventricular failure
    (D) development of a ventricular aneurysm

2. Based on the preceding information, what would be the best treatment to improve the symptoms?

    (A) oxygen therapy
    (B) dobutamine therapy
    (C) dopamine therapy
    (D) nitroprusside therapy

Questions 3 and 4 refer to the following scenario.

A 42-year-old female is in your unit following a motor vehicle accident and subsequent exploratory laporatomy. She sustained a fractured left femur, a lacerated liver, and pulmonary contusions. She is currently awake and oriented. She is receiving assisted ventilation in the AMV (assist/control) mode. Her chest x ray reveals a large left posterior lobe contusion. On postoperative day 2, her urine output decreases to 10 cc/h. The following urine and blood electrolyte information is available:

Na+	148
K+	4.4
Cl−	101
HCO_3^-	21
creatinine	3.1
BUN	64
urinary Na+	11
urinary osmolality	912

3. Based on the preceding information, what is the likely cause of the decreased urine output?

   (A) prerenal azotemia
   (B) acute tubular necrosis
   (C) acute renal failure
   (D) postrenal obstruction due to rhabdomyolysis

4. Based on preceding information, what is the most likely treatment to improve the urine output?

   (A) renal-dose dopamine
   (B) loop diuretic, e.g., Lasix
   (C) proximal tubular diuretic, e.g., mannitol
   (D) fluid bolus of normal saline

Questions 5 and 6 refer to the following scenario.

A 33-year-old male is in your unit following a fall from a second-floor balcony. He has a fractured skull and right pneumothorax. He has developed acute respiratory failure, possibly secondary to ARDS (adult respiratory distress syndrome). He has a fiber optic catheter in place to monitor his ICP (intracranial pressure). Due to refractory hypoxemia, the physician requests that the PEEP (positive end expiratory pressure) be increased to 10 cm H_2O from 5 cm H_2O. The patient manifests the following changes in vital signs after the addition of the PEEP:

	BEFORE **PEEP**	AFTER **PEEP**
blood pressure	104/66	100/62
pulse	92	88

ICP	10	17
PaO$_2$	54	76
PaCO$_2$	27	29

5. Based on the preceding information, what was the effect of the PEEP addition on cerebral oxygenation?

    (A) Oxygenation has improved based on the increased PaO$_2$.
    (B) There is no change since the PaCO$_2$ did not fall.
    (C) Oxygenation is unchanged based on the similar blood pressures.
    (D) Oxygenation has worsened due to the drop in cerebral perfusion pressure.

6. Which therapy is most likely to reduce the ICP for a short-term benefit?

    (A) a reduction in the PaCO$_2$
    (B) increasing the PaO$_2$
    (C) increasing the MAP (mean arterial pressure)
    (D) adding DDAVP (desmopressin acetate)

7. In the following ECG (electrocardiogram), what is the most significant abnormality?

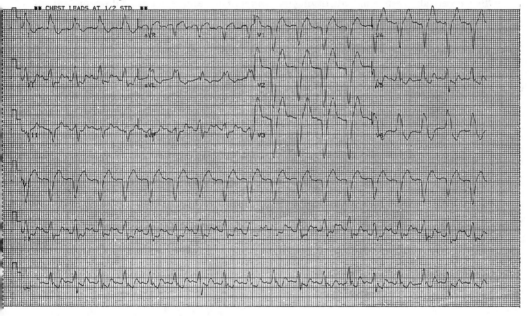

    (A) left bundle branch block
    (B) anterior MI (myocardial infarction)
    (C) posterior hemiblock
    (D) inferior wall ischemia

8. Which of the following tests is helpful in distinguishing acute renal failure from prerenal azotemia?

   (A) fractional excretion of sodium
   (B) BUN levels
   (C) creatinine levels
   (D) serum potassium values

9. Which of the following sets of blood gas values reflects a respiratory acidosis with a compensating metabolic alkalosis?

	(A)	(B)	(C)	(D)
pH	7.22	7.37	7.52	7.35
$PaCO_2$	63	36	28	62
PaO_2	65	88	75	70
HCO_3^-	24	25	30	32

Questions 10 and 11 refer to the following scenario.

A 61-kg, 32-year-old female is admitted to your unit following an acute episode of unresponsive asthma. Upon physical examination, she has generalized wheezing throughout both lung fields. She is short of breath and appears very anxious. In the emergency room, she has received 0.9 mg of subcutaneous epinephrine and a loading dose of 300 mg of aminophylline. Analysis of the first set of blood gases obtained from her in the unit reveals the following:

pH	7.44
$PaCO_2$	32
PaO_2	91
HCO_3^-	25
FIO_2	0.40

10. Based on the preceding information, which of the following treatments might be helpful in improving her clinical symptoms?

    I. corticosteroids
    II. beta stimulants
    III. incentive spirometry
       (A) I and II
       (B) I and III
       (C) II and III
       (D) I, II, and III

11. After six hours in the intensive care unit, the patient appears less anxious and is now somewhat drowsy. Her wheezing is still generalized, although it is now less intense. Analysis of her repeat blood gases indicates the following:

pH	7.32
$Paco_2$	49
Pao_2	77
HCO_3^-	25
FIO_2	0.30

Based on the preceding information, which condition is likely to be developing?

(A) She is improving based on the reduction in wheezing.
(B) She is improving based on the increased $Paco_2$.
(C) She is worsening based on the developing respiratory acidosis.
(D) There is a slight worsening due to the reduction in the Pao_2.

Questions 12 and 13 refer to the following scenario.

A 23-year-old male is in the intensive care unit following a gunshot wound to the right chest. Postoperatively, he has left posterior and anterior chest tubes. He has a three-chamber closed-chest drainage system (e.g., Pleuravac) for both air and fluid drainage. The physician requests that 20-cm H_2O suction be applied. The patient presently has bubbling in the suction control chamber, although the water seal chamber does not bubble.

12. Based on the preceding information, does the patient have a current pleural air leak?

(A) yes
(B) no
(C) As long as bubbling exists in the suction control chamber, a pleural leak is likely.
(D) It is not possible to identify a pleural leak in a three-chamber closed-chest drainage system.

13. A radiology technician calls you into a patient's room. It seems that, while maneuvering the chest x ray machine near the bed, he knocked the chest unit down and ran over it, causing a leak in the water seal chamber. When you come into the room, you can see that no fluid remains in the water seal chamber. At this point what should you do?

(A) immediately clamp the chest tube and notify the physician
(B) leave the tube open to air and call the physician
(C) call the radiology department to report the technician
(D) place the end of the chest tube into a sterile water container and replace the chest unit

14. Following an angioplasty, a 55-year-old male returns to the coronary care unit. Which of the following measures would be appropriate within the next eight hours?

   I. bedrest
   II. application of pressure over the insertion site
   III. monitoring for reperfusion dysrhythmias

     (A) I and II
     (B) I and III
     (C) II and III
     (D) I, II, and III

15. Which of the following are common reperfusion dysrhythmias following thrombolytic therapy?

   I. ventricular ectopy
   II. bradycardias
   III. atrial fibrillation/flutter

     (A) I and II
     (B) I and III
     (C) II and III
     (D) I, II, and III

Questions 16 and 17 refer to the following scenario.

A 75-year-old female has been in the intensive care unit for 15 days following surgery for a fractured pelvis suffered in a motor vehicle accident. Her postoperative course has been complicated by acute respiratory failure. She currently is off mechanical ventilation but has been spiking intermittent temperatures. She is receiving intravenous fluids (D_5W) at a rate of 75 cc/h. Her enteral feeding has been stopped for the past 48 hours due to a potential ileus. The following laboratory information is available:

Na^+	132
K^+	3.6
Cl^-	102
HCO_3^-	23
albumin	2.8
white blood cells	5100
segmented neutrophils	75%
banded neutrophils	10%
monocytes	10%
lymphocytes	5%

16. Based on the preceding information, approximately how many calories is she receiving?

(A) <200 kcal
(B) 300 to 500 kcal
(C) 700 to 900 kcal
(D) >900 kcal

17. Based on the preceding laboratory findings, which of the data are indicative of nutritional insufficiency?

   I. Na$^+$ of 132
  II. albumin of 2.8
 III. total lymphocytes of 255
     (A) I and II
     (B) I and III
     (C) II and III
     (D) I, II, and III

Questions 18 and 19 refer to the following scenario.

A 56-year-old male is in your unit following a motor vehicle accident. He sustained a fractured right humerus and a ruptured spleen. He is not responsive following surgery. He is receiving assisted ventilation in the IMV (intermittent mandatory ventilation) mode. He currently has the following vital signs:

blood pressure	96/56
pulse	125
respiratory rate	22
temperature	39°C

The physician believes that the patient may be developing hypovolemia secondary to the increased heart rate and reduced blood pressure.

18. Based on the preceding information, which condition is likely to be developing?

     (A) hypovolemia as suggested by the physician
     (B) inflammation-induced tachycardia secondary to the surgery
     (C) tachycardia secondary to infection
     (D) left ventricular failure

19. Given the above temperature, which therapy is necessary?

     (A) No therapy is necessary.
     (B) administer antipyretics
     (C) cooling blanket
     (D) ice packets to the axilla

Questions 20 and 21 refer to the following scenario.

A 73-year-old male is admitted to your unit from an oncology division. He has an admitting diagnosis of possible sepsis secondary to an unknown infectious source. His vital signs and laboratory data are listed below:

blood pressure	102/70
pulse	126
temperature	38.7°C
respiratory rate	30
white blood cells	3300
segmented neutrophils	55
banded neutrophils	10
lymphocytes	25
monocytes	7
eosinophils	1
basophils	1

20. Based on the preceding information, is the total granulocyte level abnormal?

(A) yes, based on the total number of segmented neutrophils
(B) no, based on the normal total white count
(C) yes, based on the abnormal number of lymphocytes
(D) no, based on the segmented/banded neutrophil ratio remaining in normal proportion

21. Which of the following aspects of the differential are abnormal?

I. segmented neutrophils
II. lymphocytes
III. monocytes
(A) I and II
(B) I and III
(C) II and III
(D) I, II, and III

22. A lateral wall MI (myocardial infarction) is most likely to involve which coronary artery?

(A) right coronary
(B) left main coronary
(C) left anterior descending
(D) circumflex

23. A 76-year-old female is in your unit with the diagnosis of CHF (congestive heart failure). The physician inserts a pulmonary artery catheter to aid in assessment of therapeutic treatments. One of the therapies she selects is dobutamine. With the addition of dobutamine to the treatment regime, which of the following changes in parameters would you expect to see if the therapy is successful?

   I. increase in pulmonary artery pressure
   II. reduction in PCWP (pulmonary capillary wedge pressure)
   III. increase in stroke volume

     (A) I and II
     (B) I and III
     (C) II and III
     (D) I, II, and III

24. A patient with the diagnosis of COPD (chronic obstructive pulmonary disease) is admitted to your unit with acute shortness of breath. Upon auscultation, you note that he has generalized crackles. Based on the presence of crackles and shortness of breath, the physician orders 20 mg of Lasix. Is this request appropriate?

     (A) yes, the presence of crackles suggests fluid overload
     (B) yes, due to the combined diuretic and bronchodilator effect of Lasix
     (C) no, since Lasix is a beta antagonist that may promote bronchoconstriction in addition to its diuretic effect
     (D) Not enough information is available to justify the use of Lasix since crackles may be due to airway disease, not fluid overload.

25. A 61-year-old male is in your unit postoperatively for a small bowel resection secondary to cancer. During his fifth postoperative day, he develops a small amount of hematemesis. The physician diagnoses the bleeding as originating from a potential stress ulcer. Which of the following might be effective therapies for treating this type of condition?

   I. raniditine
   II. cimetidine
   III. antacids

     (A) I and II
     (B) I and III
     (C) II and III
     (D) I, II, and III

26. A clinical specialist in your unit tells you that a new admission has a potential anterior septal MI (myocardial infarction). Which ECG leads would you examine to assess this type of injury pattern?

   (A) I, aVL
   (B) II, III, aVF
   (C) V_1 to V_4
   (D) V_5, V_6

27. Which ECG monitoring lead is most likely to detect a right bundle branch block?

   (A) II
   (B) aVF
   (C) MCL_1
   (D) $MCLr_3$

Questions 28 and 29 refer to the following scenario.

A 45-year-old male is admitted to your unit following an emergent repair of a perforated gastric ulcer. On his third postoperative day, he develops shortness of breath and a temperature elevation to 38.9°C. He is started on broad-spectrum, triple antibiotic coverage and antipyretics as indicated. His condition does not improve over the next 24 hours and he develops hypotension (blood pressure 88/58) and tachycardia (pulse 122). The physician believes that he is entering septic shock.

28. Based on the preceding information, which therapies would be useful in supporting the hypotension due to septic shock?

   I. nicardipine
   II. dopamine in levels exceeding 5 mcg/kg per min
   III. fluid bolus with normal saline
      (A) I and II
      (B) I and III
      (C) II and III
      (D) I, II, and III

29. Which of the following have been proposed as potential mediators in controlling the clinical effects of sepsis and may be effective in improving the clinical status of this patient?

   I. ibuprofen
   II. phenylephrine (Neosynephrine)
   III. naloxone (Narcan)
      (A) I and II
      (B) I and III
      (C) II and III
      (D) I, II, and III

Questions 30 and 31 refer to the following scenario.

A 71-year-old male is admitted to your unit with shortness of breath, orthopnea, and progressive reduction in exercise tolerance. He states he has "never been to a doctor." His lung sounds demonstrate crackles in most of his posterior lobes. A pulse oximeter indicates a value of 0.89. A pulmonary artery catheter is placed to help identify the origin of the shortness of breath. The following data are available:

blood pressure	118/70
pulse	110
respiratory rate	28
temperature	37.1°C
CI	2.2
SI	20
PA	36/22
PCWP	20
CVP	6

30. Based on the preceding information, which condition is likely to be developing?

    (A) left ventricular failure
    (B) primary pulmonary hypertension
    (C) sepsis
    (D) noncardiogenic pulmonary edema

31. Which therapy would most likely improve his symptoms?

    (A) oxygen therapy
    (B) Lasix
    (C) dopamine
    (D) gentamicin

Questions 32 and 33 refer to the following scenario.

A 32-year-old male construction worker is admitted to your unit following a fall from a scaffold. He suffered an epidural hematoma, which was surgically evacuated. He has a fiber optic ICP (intracranial pressure) monitor in place. Currently, he is responsive to pain and has a Glasgow Coma Score of 10. His vital signs and laboratory data are as follows:

blood pressure	122/82
pulse	66
respiratory rate	17
intracranial pressure	11

SMA6

Na$^+$	135
K$^+$	3.9
Cl$^-$	101
HCO$_3$$^-$	24
glucose	110
creatinine	1.1

ARTERIAL BLOOD GASES

pH	7.41
Pao$_2$	89
Paco$_2$	38
FIO$_2$	0.40

During your shift, he becomes less responsive; his Glasgow Coma Score decreases to 6. His current vital signs and laboratory data are as follows:

blood pressure	98/56
pulse	84
respiratory rate	25
intracranial pressure	14

SMA6

Na$^+$	137
K$^+$	3.8
Cl$^-$	100
HCO$_3$$^-$	24
glucose	99
creatinine	1.1

ARTERIAL BLOOD GASES

pH	7.39
Pao$_2$	76
Paco$_2$	35
FIO$_2$	0.40

32. Based on the preceding information, what is the most likely reason for the change in level of consciousness?

(A) change in blood glucose
(B) increase in ICP
(C) reduction in cerebral perfusion pressure
(D) reduction in Pao$_2$

33. What would be the most effective therapy for improving the level of consciousness?

(A) administration of 50 cc of $D_{50}W$

(B) administration of an osmotic diuretic (e.g., mannitol)

(C) increase the MAP (mean arterial pressure) (e.g., with dopamine)

(D) increase the FIO_2 to 0.50

Questions 34 and 35 refer to the following scenario.

A 78-year-old female is in the intensive care unit following a change in level of consciousness. Her head CT (computed tomography) scan demonstrates a large subdural bleed. This is her third day in the unit. Currently, she is responsive only to painful stimuli. Her current vital signs and laboratory data are as follows:

blood pressure	144/84
pulse	85
respiratory rate	21
temperature	37.4°C
fluid intake	3100
fluid output	6340
urinary osmolality	288
serum osmolality	324
Na^+	152

34. Based on the preceding information, which condition is likely to be developing?

(A) SIADH (syndrome of inappropriate secretion of antidiuretic hormone)

(B) myxedema coma

(C) hyperthyroidism

(D) diabetes insipidus

35. Which of the following is most likely to be an effective treatment for this condition?

(A) DDAVP (desmopressin acetate)

(B) thyroxine

(C) 500 cc D_5W

(D) propylthiouracil

36. A 42-year-old male is in your unit following a farm accident in which his chest was crushed by a tractor. He currently is intubated and is on mechanical ventilation. He has been unresponsive to oxygen therapy and PEEP (positive end expiratory pressure). His peak airway pressures are elevated (60 cm H_2O). The physician decides to add PCIRV (pressure control inverse ratio ventilation). He states that this will reduce the patient's peak airway pressure and also allow for the reduction in PEEP. How can PCIRV raise the PaO_2 and SaO_2 if peak airway pressures and PEEP are reduced?

   (A) by increasing pleural pressures
   (B) by increasing mean airway pressures
   (C) by augmenting pulmonary blood flow
   (D) through a reduction in the ventilation/perfusion ratio

Questions 37 and 38 refer to the following scenario,

A 32-year-old male with a history of bisexual social behavior is admitted to your unit from the emergency room with the diagnosis of shortness of breath of unknown origin. The emergency room physician has made a potential diagnosis of *Pneumocystis carinii* pneumonia as one of the conditions that must be ruled out. The patient is currently short of breath and requires an FIO_2 of 0.50 via face mask. On 50% oxygen, his SpO_2 is 0.90. He informs you that this is his first hospitalization involving difficulty in breathing.

37. Based on this information, which body fluids should be considered potentially dangerous?

   I. blood
   II. sputum
   III. urine
      (A) I and II
      (B) I and III
      (C) II and III
      (D) I, II, and III

38. Which of the following therapies may help treat this condition?

   I. pentamidine
   II. trimethaphan (Septra)
   III. imipenem
      (A) I and II
      (B) I and III
      (C) II and III
      (D) I, II, and III

39. Which of the following therapies has been shown to be of NO benefit in improving the clinical course of patients with sepsis?

(A) fluid bolus
(B) vasopressors
(C) inotropes
(D) steroids

40. A 56-year-old female is in your unit with the diagnosis of sepsis secondary to a urinary tract infection. She currently has the following vital signs:

blood pressure	94/58
pulse	118
respiratory rate	34
temperature	39°C

Although supportive treatments exist to help treat her symptoms, curative therapies for sepsis are limited. Which of the following therapies may be potentially successful in curing the sepsis in patients such as this one?

I. antibiotics
II. monoclonal antibodies
III. ibuprofen

(A) I
(B) II
(C) III
(D) I, II, and III

41. If the cardiac output falls secondary to hypovolemia, what is the compensatory mechanism that serves to maintain the blood pressure?

(A) increase in preload
(B) increase in systemic vascular resistance
(C) decrease in afterload
(D) increase in blood viscosity

42. With the addition of PEEP (positive end expiratory pressure) and other forms of positive pressure ventilatory assistance, the potential exists to reduce the cardiac output. What is the mechanism for the reduction in cardiac output with these therapies?

(A) increased mean airway pressures decrease thoracic blood flow
(B) through stimulation of the atrial natriuretic effect
(C) through resisting the exit of airflow at the bronchial level, thereby causing a worsening of the intrapulmonary shunt
(D) positive pressure ventilation blocks the natural passive return of blood to the heart

43. A 57-year-old male is admitted to your unit with an acute exacerbation of CHF (congestive heart failure). In order to reduce the symptoms of CHF, the physician elects to administer preload-reducing agents. Which of the following would be considered preload reducing therapies?

  I. nitroglycerine
  II. Lasix
  III. morphine

    (A) I and II
    (B) I and III
    (C) II and III
    (D) I, II, and III

44. A 31-year-old female is admitted to your unit with the diagnosis of acute gastrointestinal bleeding. She has a history of esophageal varices secondary to alcohol abuse. Which of the following are potential therapies to treat esophageal varices?

  I. raniditine
  II. intravenous vasopressin
  III. Sengstaken-Blakemore tube

    (A) I and II
    (B) I and III
    (C) II and III
    (D) I, II, and III

45. Hepatitis B is transmitted through which of the following media?

  I. blood
  II. saliva
  III. sperm

    (A) I and II
    (B) I and III
    (C) II and III
    (D) I, II, and III

46. Which of the following are considered to improve long-term survival after an MI (myocardial infarction)?

  I. aspirin
  II. beta blockers
  III. prophylactic antidysrhythmia (antiarrhythmia) agents

    (A) I and II
    (B) I and III
    (C) II and III
    (D) I, II, and III

Questions 47 and 48 refer to the following scenario.

A 67-year-old female is admitted to your unit with the diagnosis of hypotension of unknown origin. She is currently unresponsive but is breathing spontaneously and is not intubated. Breath sounds are clear, urine output is 15 cc in eight hours, and her skin is cool. A pulmonary artery (Swan-Ganz) catheter is inserted to aid the interpretation of the situation. The following data are available:

blood pressure	86/54
pulse	118
respiratory rate	30
temperature	37.3
CI	1.9
SI	16
PA	24/10
PCWP	6
CVP	3

47. Based on the preceding information, which condition is likely to be developing?

    (A) left ventricular failure
    (B) biventricular failure (CHF; congestive heart failure)
    (C) sepsis
    (D) hypovolemia

48. What would the most likely therapy for this condition include?

    (A) fluid bolus
    (B) dobutamine
    (C) dopamine
    (D) Lasix

49. Which of the following is the most common cause of a reduction in the arterial PO_2?

    (A) reduced barometric pressure
    (B) increased $PaCO_2$ levels
    (C) anatomic shunt
    (D) increased intrapulmonary shunt

50. Multisystem organ failure (MSOF) can affect any organ. Which of the following are the most commonly affected organs?

   I. liver
  II. kidney
 III. lungs

    (A) I and II
    (B) I and III
    (C) II and III
    (D) I, II, and III

Questions 51 and 52 refer to the following scenario.

A 43-year-old male is admitted to your unit with chest pain following an episode during a game of racketball. The chest pain has been present for about 90 minutes and has not been relieved by rest or position changes. His ECG demonstrates ST elevation in leads II, III, and aVF. No Q waves are present.

51. Based on the preceding information, which condition is likely to be developing?

    (A) subendocardial MI (myocardial infarction)
    (B) epicardial ischemia
    (C) inferior wall MI
    (D) Prinzmetal's angina

52. Which therapy is it most important to initiate at this time?

    (A) oxygen therapy
    (B) thrombolytic treatment
    (C) inotropic therapy (dobutamine)
    (D) afterload reduction

53. Prinzmetal's angina differs from most forms of angina in which characteristic?

   I. ST segment elevation
  II. persistent chest pain
 III. elevation of cardiac isoenzymes

    (A) I and II
    (B) I and III
    (C) II and III
    (D) I, II, and III

54. In conditions such as left ventricular failure and ARDS (adult respiratory distress syndrome), an increase in extravascular lung water occurs. What is the primary mechanism that protects alveolar function during any condition that causes an increase in extravascular lung water?

(A) increase in pulmonary interstitial osmotic pressure
(B) thickening of the alveolar membrane
(C) increase in mean alveolar pressure
(D) increase in pulmonary lymphatic drainage

55. Use of a pH probe at the tip of a nasogastric tube is thought to aid in monitoring the passage of the tube through the gastrointestinal tract. What factors make this strategy possible?

   I. the pH of the stomach is highly acidic
  II. the pH of the duodenum is alkaline
 III. the pH of the jejenum is neutral
   (A) I and II
   (B) I and III
   (C) II and III
   (D) I, II, and III

56. Which of the following substrates serve as the primary energy source for cerebral metabolism?

(A) proteins
(B) fats
(C) carbohydrates
(D) ketones

57. A 63-year-old male is in your unit after being transferred from the emergency room. He was found lying unresponsive in his apartment by his neighbor. His admitting diagnosis is reduced level of consciousness of unknown origin. Based on this diagnosis, which of the following would be considered as potential causes of the decreased level of consciousness?

   I. blood glucose level of less than 60
  II. cerebral perfusion pressure of less than 60 mm Hg
 III. urinary sodium level of less than 20 meq
   (A) I and II
   (B) I and III
   (C) II and III
   (D) I, II, and III

58. Clinical estimation of left ventricular preload is assumed to be possible by utilizing which parameter?

(A) central venous pressure
(B) PCWP (pulmonary capillary wedge pressure)
(C) left ventricular stroke work index
(D) coronary sinus pressure

59. Cyanosis may be an unreliable sign of arterial oxygenation. Why can cyanosis be misleading?

I. Cyanosis is only present in patients with a reduced cardiac output.
II. Cyanosis reflects capillary, not necessarily arterial, oxyhemoglobin levels.
III. Bluish discoloration is visible only with adequate hemoglobin levels.

(A) I and II
(B) I and III
(C) II and III
(D) I, II, and III

Questions 60 and 61 refer to the following scenario.

A 65-year-old male is in your unit after developing hypotension on the floor. He had femoral-popliteal bypass surgery four days earlier and was doing well until yesterday. He began to complain of generalized malaise with the following vital signs:

blood pressure	122/78
pulse	110
respiratory rate	27
temperature	38.1°C

His wound site is reddened but has no drainage. This morning, he was less well oriented and was hypotensive (blood pressure 88/54, pulse 114), prompting a transfer to the unit. He does not complain of any discomfort or shortness of breath. His lung sounds are clear and he has a pulse oximeter value of 0.99. A flow-directed pulmonary artery catheter is inserted to assist in the assessment of the cause of the hypotension. The following data are available from the pulmonary artery catheter:

CO	10.5
CI	6.0
PA	22/11
PCWP	8
CVP	2

60. Based on the preceding information, which condition is likely to be developing?

(A) bleeding into the postoperative wound site
(B) left ventricular failure
(C) hypovolemia
(D) sepsis

61. Which treatment is likely to be instituted in this scenario?

(A) exploratory opening and draining of the surgical wound
(B) broad-spectrum antibiotics
(C) dobutamine at 5 mcg/kg per min
(D) fluid bolus with D_5W at 100 cc/h

62. Which of the following characterizes ARDS (adult respiratory distress syndrome)?

I. resistive hypoxemia
II. "white-out" appearance on the chest x ray
III. cyanosis
    (A) I and II
    (B) I and III
    (C) II and III
    (D) I, II, and III

63. A 76-year-old male is admitted with CHF (congestive heart failure) secondary to systemic hypertension. The physician states that she wants initially to attempt afterload manipulation to aid the CHF. Which of the following may alter afterload favorably to improve the condition?

I. nicardipine
II. labetalol
III. enalapril
    (A) I and II
    (B) I and III
    (C) II and III
    (D) I, II, and III

64. In the patient with a cardiomyopathy, which of the following treatment options are likely to improve cardiac output?

I. dobutamine
II. angiotension converting enzyme inhibitors
III. dopamine
    (A) I and II
    (B) I and III
    (C) II and III
    (D) I, II, and III

65. What is the most likely reason for increased cardiac output in a septic patient?

(A) decreased venous return
(B) decreased systemic vascular resistance
(C) increased sympathetic catecholamine stimulation
(D) decreased parasympathetic stimulation

66. Which of the following are therapies likely to be used to treat an unknown source of sepsis?

I. gentamycin (gram-negative antibiotic)
II. fluid challenge
III. ampicillin (gram-positive antibiotic)

(A) I and II
(B) I and III
(C) II and III
(D) I, II, and III

67. At what level of oxygen is oxygen toxicity thought to develop?

(A) 30% for 4 hours
(B) 40% for 12 hours
(C) 50% for 24 hours
(D) any FIO_2 greater than room air (0.21) if exposed for more than two consecutive hours

68. Which of the following are components of cardiac output?

I. systemic vascular resistance
II. stroke volume
III. heart rate

(A) I and II
(B) I and III
(C) II and III
(D) I, II, and III

69. A 55-year-old male is admitted to your unit with the diagnosis of CHF (congestive heart failure). In order to increase his cardiac output without increasing his myocardial oxygen demand, which of the following therapies might be utilized?

I. nitroprusside
II. dobutamine
III. captopril
    (A) I and II
    (B) I and III
    (C) II and III
    (D) I, II, and III

Questions 70 and 71 refer to the following scenario.

A 66-year-old male is admitted to your unit with the diagnosis of upper gastrointestinal bleeding. He is currently jaundiced, has a distended abdomen, and appears cachectic. He has had a prior endoscopy for an earlier episode of gastrointestinal bleeding, at which time he was noted to have esophageal varices. He is confused as to time and place.

70. Based on the preceding information, which therapy is the most important to initiate to control the bleeding?

    (A) endoscopy
    (B) intravenous H_2 blockers
    (C) surgical creation of a portacaval shunt
    (D) esophageal balloon (Sengstaken-Blakemore) tube

71. Which of the following symptoms would indicate a large bleed occurring from the varices?

    I. epigastric pain
    II. hypotension
    III. tachycardia
        (A) I and II
        (B) I and III
        (C) II and III
        (D) I, II, and III

72. A 45-year-old male is in your unit with the diagnosis of acute respiratory failure secondary to refractory pneumonia. He is intubated and presently receiving an FIO_2 of 0.70 and +5 cm H_2O PEEP (positive end expiratory pressure). He is on AMV (assist/control mechanical ventilation) with a rate of 12 and a VT of 800 cc. He has the following blood gas values on these settings:

pH	7.37
$PaCO_2$	40
PaO_2	51
HCO_3^-	23

Vital signs at this time are a blood pressure of 122/78 and a pulse of 88. Based on the blood gas values, the PEEP setting is increased to 10 cm H_2O. A repeat blood gas analysis reveals the following:

pH	7.35
$PaCO_2$	38
PaO_2	67
HCO_3^-	26

Vital signs now show a blood pressure of 104/62 and a pulse of 109. Based on the information provided, has the change in PEEP been effective in improving oxygen delivery?

(A) no, based on the change in blood pressure and heart rate
(B) yes, based on the change in PaO_2
(C) unable to tell without a pulse oximeter reading
(D) unable to tell without a hemoglobin level

73. If a pulse oximeter reading (SpO_2) is 0.96, what is the likely value for the actual oxyhemoglobin value (SaO_2), assuming no unusual conditions exist that might interfere with light absorption?

(A) 0.90
(B) 0.93
(C) 0.96
(D) 0.99

74. Which of the following is the most common cause for an MI (myocardial infarction)?

(A) thrombosis around an atherosclerotic plaque
(B) excessive myocardial oxygen consumption
(C) obstruction of the coronary artery by lipid accumulation
(D) decreased diastolic filling pressures

75. Which of the following is considered the most accurate measure for determining whether an MI (myocardial infarction) has occurred?

(A) 12-lead ECG
(B) cardiac isoenzymes
(C) two-dimensional echocardiography
(D) coronary angiography

Questions 76 and 77 refer to the following scenario.

A 71-year-old male is admitted to the intensive care unit with hypotension of unknown origin. He currently has a fiber optic pulmonary artery catheter in place to determine the origin of the hypotension. At 1800, he is unresponsive with a Glasgow Coma Score of 4. His vital signs and pulmonary artery catheter reveal the following information:

blood pressure	102/68
pulse	101
CO	3.9
CI	2.4
PA	42/22
PCWP	14
CVP	12
SvO_2	0.56

The physician requests that dobutamine be added to his treatment. One hour after the administration of the dobutamine, a repeat set of hemodynamics reveals the following:

blood pressure	104/66
pulse	106
CO	4.4
CI	2.6
PA	40/23
PCWP	14
CVP	13
SvO_2	.56

76. Based on the preceding information, why did the increase in cardiac output not produce an improvement in the SvO_2?

    (A) SvO_2 reflects oxygenation, not the adequacy of hemodynamics.
    (B) The increase in cardiac output was not adequate to meet cellular demands for oxygen.
    (C) The oxygen consumption decreased.
    (D) SvO_2 reflects venous oxygen, not arterial flow, which is what is measured by cardiac output values.

77. Based on the preceding information, which therapy would most likely be effective in improving cellular oxygenation?

    (A) oxygen
    (B) increasing dobutamine
    (C) adding norepinephrine (Levophed)
    (D) adding bronchodilators

78. A 44-year-old male is admitted to your unit with the diagnosis of hypotension of unknown origin, although sepsis from a possible pneumonia is a potential cause. He has no complaints of discomfort other than a persistent cough and low-grade temperature (37.6°C). His lung sounds are clear except for a slight increase in sound in the left lingular area. His urine output is low and appears concentrated. Urinary electrolytes are not available yet. A pulmonary artery (Swan-Ganz) catheter is inserted to aid in assessment. The following data are available from the catheter:

CO	9.2
CI	5.3
PA	19/10
PCWP	7
CVP	1

While you are discussing these data with a new orientee, she states that they suggest that the patient is hypovolemic, not septic. Which data would help differentiate sepsis from hypovolemia and thereby help you explain to the new nurse how to interpret the information?

    I. concentrated urine
    II. clear lung sounds
    III. high cardiac output and stroke volumes with low PCWP

        (A) I
        (B) II
        (C) III
        (D) I, II, and III

Questions 79 and 80 refer to the following scenario.

A 78-year-old male is in your unit with potential multisystem organ failure. He currently is on mechanical ventilation with an FIO_2 of 0.70, and a PEEP of +8. The nurse on the prior shift cautioned you that this patient's heart rate drops during suctioning. During your initial suctioning, you note that his heart rate decreases from 83 to 45 bpm.

79. What is the likely cause of this reduction in heart rate?

    (A) reduction in PaO_2
    (B) reduction in $PaCO_2$
    (C) phrenic nerve stimulation
    (D) vagal nerve stimuation

80. Which treatment would most likely prevent the decrease in heart rate?

(A) hyperoxygenation
(B) hyperventilation
(C) use of lower suction pressures
(D) administration of 0.5 mg atropine

Questions 81 and 82 refer to the following scenario.

A 76-year-old female is admitted to your unit from the emergency room with unexplained unresponsiveness. Her husband states that she had not been "feeling well" for the past few days but that this morning she became short of breath and confused. He called emergency medical services, who brought her to the emergency room. Upon admission to the intensive care unit, she was unresponsive and intubated, with admission blood pressure of 76/44 and heart rate of 117. Analysis of her blood gases reveals the following:

pH	7.30
$PaCO_2$	21
PaO_2	63
HCO_3^-	16
FIO_2	0.70

A pulmonary artery catheter was inserted to help assess her condition. The catheter supplied the following data:

CI	1.5
PA	42/27
PCWP	25
CVP	15

81. Based on the preceding information, which condition is likely to be present?

   (A) hypovolemic shock
   (B) noncardiogenic shock
   (C) cardiogenic shock
   (D) neurogenic shock

82. Which therapy is most likely to help improve her clinical condition?

   I. dopamine
   II. dobutamine
   III. Lasix
      (A) I and II
      (B) I and III
      (C) II and III
      (D) I, II, and III

83. A 85-year-old female in your unit with possible pulmonary emobolism develops shortness of breath and hypotension (blood pressure 82/52) during your shift. Based on these symptoms, the physician is concerned with tissue oxygenation. Which of the following parameters would be good indicators of cellular hypoxia?

I. arterial blood gas values specifically PaO_2 levels
II. SvO_2 values
III. lactate levels

(A) I and II
(B) I and III
(C) II and III
(D) I

84. Systemic hypertension produces which type of effect on the left ventricle?

I. dilation of the chamber
II. thickening of the ventricular muscle wall
III. increase in ventricular end diastolic pressure

(A) I and II
(B) I and III
(C) II and III
(D) I, II, and III

Questions 85 and 86 refer to the following scenario.

A 23-year-old female is admitted to your unit with unresponsiveness of unknown origin. Her roommate states that, while she was away for the weekend, her friend had stayed home. When she returned, she found her friend unresponsive. Currently, her skin is warm to the touch and she responds only to painful stimuli. Her urine output is about 17 cc for the past hour. She is scheduled for a head CAT scan and has the following laboratory data:

Na^+	148
K^+	4.9
Cl^-	111
HCO_3^-	14
glucose	655
plasma osmolality	344
pH	7.19
$PaCO_2$	28
PaO_2	88

85. Based on the preceding information, which condition is likely to be developing?

(A) diabetes insipidus
(B) diabetic hyperosmolar coma
(C) diabetic ketoacidosis
(D) exacerbation of acute renal failure

86. Which of the following therapies would most likely be effective in treating this condition?

(A) normal saline fluid bolus
(B) initiation of an insulin drip
(C) sodium bicarbonate drip
(D) fluid bolus of D_5W

87. Which of the following are potential causes for the development of giant A waves in a CVP (central venous pressure) or PCWP (pulmonary capillary wedge pressure) waveform?

   I. noncompliant atrium
  II. mitral or tricuspid regurgitation
 III. pulmonary or systemic hypertension
     (A) I and II
     (B) I and III
     (C) II and III
     (D) I, II, and III

88. A 81-year-old male is admitted with the diagnosis of right ventricular MI (myocardial infarction). In order to assess therapy, right ventricular preload will need to be monitored. Which of the following parameters will therefore need to be measured?

(A) pulmonary vascular resistance
(B) right ventricular stroke work index
(C) CVP (central venous pressure)
(D) PCWP (pulmonary capillary wedge pressure)

89. Which of the following statements best describes the difference between AMV (assisted mandatory or assist/control ventilation) and PSV (pressure support ventilation)?

   I. AMV is able to deliver larger tidal volumes than PSV.
  II. AMV gives more consistent tidal volumes than PSV.
 III. AMV tidal volumes are volume limited, not pressure limited like those of PSV.
     (A) I and II
     (B) I and III
     (C) II and III
     (D) I, II, and III

90. Which of the following are the major factors in regulating blood pressure?

> **I.** cardiac output
> **II.** systemic vascular resistance
> **III.** ventricular wall tension
>> **(A)** I and II
>> **(B)** I and III
>> **(C)** II and III
>> **(D)** I, II, and III

91. Reverse isolation frequently is ineffective in preventing infections for which of the following reasons?

> **I.** autoinfection from resident pathogens
> **II.** failure of the staff to use adequate precautions
> **III.** the presence of multiple infectious agents in the hospital setting
>> **(A)** I and II
>> **(B)** I and III
>> **(C)** II and III
>> **(D)** I, II, and III

92. In the septic cascade, a variety of agents are released that alter vascular reactivity. All of the following cause vasoconstriction and reduce capillary blood flow but one. Which of the following is a vasodilator and may improve capillary blood flow in sepsis?

> **(A)** tumor necrosing factor
> **(B)** interleukin 1
> **(C)** thromboxane A_2
> **(D)** prostaglandin E_1

93. A 51-year-old female is admitted to your unit with the diagnosis of acute inferior wall MI (myocardial infarction). Which type of dysrhythmia is she potentially likely to develop?

> **(A)** second-degree type 1 heart block
> **(B)** second-degree type 2 heart block
> **(C)** third-degree heart block
> **(D)** idioventricular escape rhythm

94. A 67-year-old female is admitted to your unit following a cardiopulmonary arrest on a step-down unit. When she is admitted to the unit, she is unresponsive to verbal stimuli but, when the sole of her foot is stroked, she demonstrates a positive extensor plantar (Babinski) reflex. Based on this response, what type of neurologic condition is present?

(A) upper motor neuron impairment
(B) lower motor neuron impairment
(C) left cerebral infarct
(D) cerebellar infarct

95. When reading a pulmonary artery pressure waveform, what is the best location at which to avoid respiratory artifact?

(A) end inspiration
(B) end QRS complex
(C) during the trough (lowest point) of a spontaneous breath
(D) end expiration

96. Which of the following physical signs are consistent with left ventricular failure?

I. S_3 or gallop rhythm
II. dependent crackles in the lungs
III. systemic hypotension
    (A) I and II
    (B) I and III
    (C) II and III
    (D) I, II, and III

Questions 97 and 98 refer to the following scenario.

An 81-year-old male admitted to your unit with the diagnosis of CVA (cerebrovascular accident). He has been unresponsive since admission and the family has requested that that no aggressive measures be performed regarding resuscitation. On your shift, you note that his left pupil dilates and is unresponsive to light.

97. Based on this information, which condition is likely to be developing?

(A) uncal herniation
(B) ventricular bleeding
(C) brainstem edema
(D) medullary compression

98. Which nerve is likely to be involved in this situation?

(A) optic (cranial nerve II)
(B) oculomotor (cranial nerve III)
(C) vagal (cranial nerve X)
(D) trigeminal (cranial nerve V)

99. A 71-year-old female is in your unit following a small bowel resection. On her second postoperative day, the physician requests weaning parameters to determine if she is ready to be removed from mechanical ventilation. Which of the following tests would be indicators of successful spontaneous breathing and therefore successful weaning?

I. respiratory rate less than 30
II. minute ventilation between 5 and 10 LPM
III. peak inspiratory effort > -20 cm H_2O

   (A) I and II
   (B) I and III
   (C) II and III
   (D) I, II, and III

100. While starting an IV in a newly admitted 33-year-old male with the diagnosis of hepatitis, you accidentally stick yourself with the needle. Which type of hepatitis would you be most at risk for developing?

   (A) hepatitis A
   (B) hepatitis B
   (C) hepatitis C
   (D) hepatitis D

101. A 55-year-old male is in your unit following an episode of hypotension during surgery for a ruptured bowel. His hypotension has resolved but he continues to manifest an acidotic pH of metabolic origin. Which of the following would be suggestive of a reason for the acidosis?

   (A) anion gap >15
   (B) low $PaCO_2$ level
   (C) BUN:creatinine ratio of less than 15:1
   (D) BUN level of 35

Questions 102 and 103 refer to the following scenario.

A 66-year-old male develops third-degree heart block with a rate of 44 and a blood pressure of 86/52 after an MI (myocardial infarction). Along with this rhythm, he has occasional PVCs (premature ventricular contractions).

102. Which of the following would be considered effective therapies for this situation?

   I. lidocaine
   II. atropine
   III. isoproterenol

(A) I and II
(B) I and III
(C) II and III
(D) I, II, and III

103. Assume that the initial therapies have failed and the physician elects to place an external pacemaker. Which of the following nursing considerations present themselves with the use of the external pacemaker?

   I. potential need for sedation
   II. instruction to the patient regarding possible muscle twitching
   III. warning the patient of potential minor burning of the skin

   (A) I and II
   (B) I and III
   (C) II and III
   (D) I, II, and III

Questions 104 and 105 refer to the following scenario.

A 77-year-old female is in your unit following a fall down a flight of stairs. She suffered a fracture of her right femur and left humerus along with a ruptured spleen. Postoperatively, she is in the unit for hemodynamic stabilization before being discharged to the floor. During the first two postoperative days, her vital signs are stable, she is alert and oriented, and, besides requiring medication for pain, she is in no overt distress. During the third postoperative day, she begins to complain of shortness of breath and pain in her left chest. The pain does not change with respiration. Oxygen therapy is initiated (face mask at 30%) and sublingual nitroglycerine is given. No improvement in symptoms is noted. A stat ECG shows no ischemic changes. A blood gas analysis reveals the following:

pH	7.45
$PaCO_2$	31
PaO_2	76
HCO_3^-	24
FIO_2	0.30

Auscultation of her lungs reveals that they are clear except for a few crackles in the right posterior area.

104. Based on the preceding information, which condition is likely to be developing?

   (A) left ventricular failure
   (B) right ventricular failure
   (C) pulmonary emboli
   (D) ARDS (adult respiratory distress syndrome)

105. Based on the preceding information, which therapy is most likely to help improve her symptoms?

(A) increase the FIO_2 to 0.50
(B) use of thrombolytic therapy (e.g., tissue plasminogen activator or streptokinase)
(C) addition of heparin
(D) intravenous nitroglycerine

106. In a hypotensive patient who is normovolemic, which of the following agents could be used to raise the blood pressure?

I. dopamine
II. norepinephrine
III. phenylephrine

(A) I and II
(B) I and III
(C) II and III
(D) I, II, and III

Questions 107 and 108 refer to the following scenario.

During your shift, you notice that the urine output of a 58-year-old COPD (chronic obstructive pulmonary disease) patient decreases to 75 cc total. He has a history of pulmonary hypertension and a 45-pack-per-year history of smoking. The following information is also available to you:

Na^+	121
K^+	3.6
Cl^-	88
HCO_3^-	22
creatinine	2.0
BUN	27
osmolality	267
urinary osmolality	319
urinary Na^+	32

107. Based on the preceding information, which condition is likely to be developing?

(A) prerenal azotemia
(B) acute renal failure
(C) diabetes insipidus
(D) inappropriate secretion of antidiuretic hormone

108. Which treatment plan would you consider?

(A) vasopressin
(B) fluid bolus
(C) diuretics
(D) DDAVP (desmopressin acetate)

109. A 54-year-old male is admitted to your unit with the diagnosis of hepatic failure. Which of the following disturbances could you expect to see in a patient with this diagnosis?

  I. disturbance in glucose regulation
 II. excessive bleeding tendencies
III. low serum protein levels

  (A) I and II
  (B) I and III
  (C) II and III
  (D) I, II, and III

110. Following a motor vehicle accident, a 20-year-old female is admitted to your unit for observation. She has possible blunt chest trauma, although no overt injuries are present. In attempting to establish whether myocardial injury has occurred, which of the following tests might be useful?

  I. CPK (creatine phosphokinase) isoenzyme analysis
 II. 12-lead ECG
III. chest x ray

  (A) I and II
  (B) I and III
  (C) II and III
  (D) I, II, and III

111. Therapies designed to improve the cardiac performance in a patient with cardiomyopathy can be monitored by several measures. Which of the measures below would indicate a positive response to treatment in a patient with a cardiomyopathy?

  I. increased PCWP (pulmonary capillary wedge pressure)
 II. increased ejection fraction
III. increased left ventricular end diastolic volume

  (A) I
  (B) II
  (C) I and III
  (D) II and III

112. Which of the following tests is most diagnostic for a pulmonary embolism?

(A) arterial blood gas analysis
(B) pulmonary angiography
(C) chest x-ray
(D) ventilation/perfusion scan

113. Which of the following clinical symptoms are consistent with the diagnosis of sepsis?

I. hypo- or hyperthermia
II. tachycardia
III. warm extremities

(A) I and II
(B) I and III
(C) II and III
(D) I, II, and III

114. A 48-year-old male is admitted to your unit with the diagnosis of anterior wall MI (myocardial infarction). During your shift, he develops ventricular fibrillation and requires resuscitation. Which of the following medications would be administered during the ventricular fibrillation situation?

I. dopamine
II. epinephrine
III. lidocaine

(A) I and II
(B) I and III
(C) II and III
(D) I, II, and III

Questions 115 and 116 refer to the following scenario.

A 20-year-old female is in your unit following chemotherapy and radiation treatments for lymphoma. She currently is markedly short of breath, with the following information available:

blood pressure	98/64
pulse	133
respiratory rate	41
temperature	39
PaO_2	66
FIO_2	0.80 (face mask)
pH	7.33
$PaCO_2$	30
HCO_3^-	20
white blood cells	1800

She has crackles throughout both lung fields, a strong pulse, and warm, moist skin.

115. Based on the preceding information, which condition is likely to be developing?

   I. systemic response to immunosuppression
   II. pulmonary capillary leak syndrome
   III. left ventricular failure

   (A) I and II
   (B) I and III
   (C) II and III
   (D) I, II, and III

116. Which therapy is most likely to improve her symptoms and reduce her distress immediately?

   I. antibiotic therapy
   II. mechanical ventilation
   III. intubation and sedation

   (A) I and II
   (B) I and III
   (C) II and III
   (D) I, II, and III

Questions 117 and 118 refer to the following scenario.

A 47-year-old female is admitted to your unit following an attempted suicide through an overdose of acetaminophen and aspirin. During the initial 24 hours, she requires intubation for decreased level of consciousness. She is placed on a ventilator set to AMV (assist/control) mode with a tidal volume of 750 cc and a rate of 12. She has markedly elevated liver enzymes and develops compartment syndrome bilaterally in her lower legs. The compartment syndrome requires fasciotomy to relieve the pressure. On the second day of admission, she is alert and appears oriented. During your shift, she begins to indicate that she is having difficulty breathing. Her pulse oximeter reading changes from 0.98 to 0.86 on an FIO_2 of 0.30. The physician requests that the FIO_2 be increased to 0.50 and that a stat chest x ray be obtained. The SpO_2 changes from 0.86 to 0.89 and the chest x ray shows diffuse infiltrates throughout her lungs. The physician requests that the FIO_2 be increased to 0.70, which results in the SpO_2 changing from 0.89 to 0.90.

117. Based on the preceding information, which condition is likely to be developing?

   (A) pulmonary hemorrhage
   (B) ARDS (adult respiratory distress syndrome)
   (C) pulmonary emboli
   (D) unilateral pulmonary edema

118. Which therapy is most likely to improve the arterial hypoxemia produced by the situation?

(A) increasing the FIO_2 to 100
(B) changing from AMV to PSV (pressure support ventilation)
(C) performing a therapeutic bronchoscopy
(D) adding PEEP (positive end expiratory pressure)

119. Tissue plasminogen activators work by means of which mechanism?

(A) blocking the production of thromboxane A_2
(B) stimulating the process of fibrin degradation
(C) stimulating endothelial ion activation
(D) accelerating the release of arachidonic acid

120. Interpret the following ECG rhythm strip.

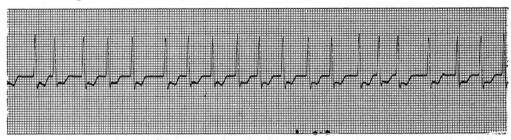

(A) atrial fibrillation
(B) sinus tachycardia with block
(C) atrial tachycardia with block
(D) atrial flutter with block

121. Which of the following test results would be indicative of chronic hepatic failure?

I. SGOT level of 458
II. alkaline phosphatase level of 352
III. bilirubin level of 35 mg/dL

(A) I and II
(B) I and III
(C) II and III
(D) I, II, and III

Questions 122 and 123 refer to the following scenario.

A 33-year-old male is admitted to your unit with complaints of progressive muscular weakness. He states that he noticed that the symptoms have "worked upward from my toes and hands to now involve my arms and legs." He has noted a persistent shortness of breath over the past 24 hours.

122. Based on the preceding information, which clinical condition is likely to be developing?

    (A) muscular dystrophy
    (B) multiple sclerosis
    (C) generalized myositis
    (D) Guillain-Barré syndrome

123. Which of the following is most likely to improve the clinical symptoms exhibited by this patient?

    (A) plasmapheresis
    (B) steroids
    (C) Dilantin
    (D) electrotherapy

Questions 124 and 125 refer to the following scenario.

A 77-year-old female is in your unit with the diagnosis of CHF (congestive heart failure). She currently is not short of breath but complains of orthopnea. She is on a 40% high-humidity face mask with an SpO_2 value of 0.95. Inspiratory crackles are present along her posterior lobe. In the hemodynamic parameters listed below, you note a change in some parameters between 0400 and 0500.

	0400	**0500**
blood pressure	100/60	102/56
pulse	110	108
respiratory rate	25	27
CI	2.4	2.3
SI	22	21
PA	39/19	43/24
PCWP	16	22
CVP	10	13

124. Based on the preceding information, has any clinically significant change in hemodynamics occurred?

(A) Yes, the pulmonary capillary wedge pressure is elevated.
(B) Yes, the stroke index has fallen.
(C) No, the changes are generally within the range seen with normal measurement error.
(D) No, the decrease in stroke index has been matched by an increase in blood pressure.

125. Based on the change in hemodynamics, what treatment would be indicated?

(A) No treatment would be indicated.
(B) dobutamine
(C) Lasix
(D) dopamine

126. Which of the following components of the immune system provide the initial response to an infection?

(A) neutrophils
(B) lymphocytes
(C) monocytes
(D) eosinophils

127. During the initial response to an antigen, one component of the immune system is responsible for stimulating the immune system to start producing antibodies. Which of the following components of the immune system stimulates antibody production?

(A) segmented neutrophils
(B) T4 lymphocytes
(C) T8 lymphocytes
(D) immunoglobulin

128. The combination therapy of dobutamine and nitroprusside is designed to improve hemodynamics by which action?

(A) increasing contractility and preload
(B) increasing afterload and contractility
(C) reducing afterload and increasing cardiac/stroke index
(D) reducing preload and increasing cardiac/stroke index

Questions 129 and 130 refer to the following scenario.

While helping a new orientee pull a patient up in bed, you notice after she lets the side rail down that the low-pressure alarm on the ventilator is activated.

129. When the low-pressure alarm is activated, what is likely to be occuring?

    (A) The patient has secretions in the endotracheal tube.
    (B) The ventilator is not meeting the expected resistance to give a breath.
    (C) The endotracheal tube is out of place.
    (D) The inspiratory time has decreased to the point that the programmed inspiratory pressure is not being met.

130. After this event, the orientee is concerned that she would not have known what to do had you not been in the room. What would be the best course of action to treat a low-pressure alarm if the cause was not immediately evident?

    (A) suction the endotracheal tube
    (B) increase the FIO_2 from the ventilator
    (C) increase the tidal volume from the ventilator and call respiratory therapy for assistance
    (D) remove the ventilator and use a manual resuscitator (e.g., Ambu bag) until assistance arrived

131. What is the maximum time after an MI (myocardial infarction) during which thrombolytics are considered still to be effective?

    (A) 1 to 2 hours
    (B) 3 to 4 hours
    (C) <6 hours
    (D) anytime within the first 24 hours

132. A 61-year-old male has a two-day history of abdominal pain with nausea and vomiting. He has intermittent chest pain that is unrelieved by nitrates, position, or rest. He has a history of CHF (congestive heart failure) and underwent a CABG (coronary artery bypass graft) two years ago. Currently he has a urine output of 15 cc/h. He has had a urine output of 200 cc over the past 24 hours. He has the following vital signs, laboratory data, and hemodynamic information:

blood pressure	88/56
pulse	114
respiratory rate	32
CO	3.7
CI	2.4
PA	20/8
PCWP	6
CVP	2
Na^+	153
K^+	3.6
Cl^-	120
HCO_3^-	19
creatinine	2.2
glucose	154
BUN	35
osmolality	320
urinary osmolality	845
urinary Na^+	34
urinary creatinine	48

Based on the preceding information, which condition is likely to be developing?

(A) prerenal azotemia from hypovolemia
(B) prerenal azotemia from left ventricular failure
(C) acute renal failure
(D) postrenal obstruction

Questions 133 and 134 refer to the following scenario.

A 41-year-old female is admitted to your unit with abdominal pain and hypotension. She states that the pain is severe and unremitting, is primarily epigastric, and "goes into my back." She has the following laboratory data:

Na^+	140
K^+	4.3
Cl^-	104
HCO_3^-	21
glucose	531
white blood cells	13,300
BUN	48
amylase	464
calcium	6.6 mg/dL

133. Based on the preceding information, which condition is likely to be developing?

    (A) hyperglycemic reaction
    (B) perforation of gastric ulcer
    (C) pancreatitis
    (D) hepatic inflammation

134. Which of the following treatments would most likely be effective in this condition?

    I. initiation of NPO (non per os; nothing by mouth) status
    II. surgical intervention
    III. administration of meperidine (Demerol) for pain relief

        (A) I and II
        (B) I and III
        (C) II and III
        (D) I, II, and III

Questions 135 and 136 refer to the following scenario.

A 34-year-old male is admitted to your unit following surgical repair of a lacerated liver from a motor vehicle accident. During your shift on postoperative day 1, his blood pressure falls from 134/84 to 88/56 and his heart rate increases from 78 to 122. His skin is cool and clammy and he denies shortness of breath, although he is slightly confused. Heart sounds are normal and lungs are clear.

135. Based on these changes, which condition is likely to be developing?

    (A) left ventricular failure
    (B) hypovolemia secondary to bleeding
    (C) parasympathetic response due to vagal stimulation
    (D) hypotension secondary to lack of protein production due to hepatic failure

136. Which of the following would be most effective in rapidly increasing the blood pressure in this situation?

    (A) dobutamine
    (B) dopamine
    (C) 500 cc of 6% Hetastarch
    (D) 500 cc of normal saline

137. During monitoring of a 63-year-old male with acute respiratory failure, you note his end tidal PCO_2 value to be 33. Assuming a normal correlation between the end tidal and arterial CO_2 exists, what would the approximate arterial PCO_2 value be if the end tidal PCO_2 was 33 mm Hg?

(A) 29
(B) 33
(C) 37
(D) 41

Questions 138 and 139 refer to the following scenario.

Following a code on a 56-year-old male, you notice that breath sounds are decreased on the left. His pulse oximeter is reading 0.98 on an FIO_2 of 0.50. The right lung has good breath sounds with a few coarse crackles. His blood pressure is 142/84 and his pulse is 94. He is currently unresponsive to verbal stimuli.

138. Based on the preceding information, which condition is likely to be present?

(A) right bronchial intubation
(B) mucous plug of the left mainstem
(C) left pneumothorax
(D) ventilator malfunction

139. Which test is most likely to detect the cause of the difference in breath sounds?

(A) arterial blood gas analysis
(B) ventilator perfusion scan
(C) chest x-ray
(D) capnography and end tidal CO_2 analysis

140. A patient is admitted to your unit with the diagnosis of low cardiac output secondary to myocardial injury. The physician elects to insert an intraaortic balloon pump (IABP) in order to improve his clinical situation. Which of the following are considered major advantages to intraaortic balloon pumping?

I. reduction in afterload
II. improvement in preload
III. improvement in coronary perfusion

(A) I and II
(B) I and III
(C) II and III
(D) I, II, and III

141. The human immunodeficiency virus (HIV) and the antirejection drug cyclosporine both act to inhibit one aspect of the immune system. Which part of the immune system is blocked by both the HIV and cyclosporine?

   (A) plasma cells
   (B) killer T cells
   (C) T4 lymphocytes
   (D) B-cell lymphocytes

142. Which of the following are considered major risk factors for the development of sepsis?

   I. sex (males develop sepsis more than females)
   II. age (>65 years)
   III. invasive procedures

   (A) I and II
   (B) I and III
   (C) II and III
   (D) I, II, and III

Questions 143 and 144 refer to the following scenario.

A 49-year-old male is in your unit following a CABG (coronary artery bypass graft). He has not responded to conventional methods to wean him from mechanical ventilation and has been in the unit for two weeks. During report, the nurse on the shift prior to yours states that she is concerned over the lack of activity and the potential for development of DVT (deep venous thrombosis).

143. Which of the following would be signs of the presence of DVT?

   I. pulmonary emboli
   II. loss of pedal pulses
   III. increased temperature in the affected leg

   (A) I and II
   (B) I and III
   (C) II and III
   (D) I, II, and III

144. Which of the following would be considered effective therapies to prevent the development of DVT?

   I. alternating compression devices on the legs
   II. aspirin
   III. active leg exercises

   (A) I and II
   (B) I and III
   (C) II and III
   (D) I, II, and III

145. Inflation of the IABP (intraaortic balloon pump) should coincide with which of the following hemodynamic events?

(A) end ventricular diastole
(B) peak V-wave point
(C) dicrotic notch
(D) anacrotic notch

146. Which of the following are unlikely to help alter the course of a patient with ARDS (adult respiratory distress syndrome)?

I. antibiotics
II. PEEP (positive end expiratory pressure)
III. steroids

(A) I and II
(B) I and III
(C) II and III
(D) I, II, and III

147. A 77-year-old female is in your unit following an episode of angina that precipitated an episode of CHF (congestive heart failure). She has a pulmonary artery catheter in place, which provides an initial set of information. A second set of hemodynamic values indicates her status following the initiation of nitroglycerine. Based on the data, was the nitroglycerine effective in improving her hemodynamics?

	INITIAL VALUES	VALUES AFTER NITROGLYCERINE
blood pressure	114/76	112/72
pulse	106	92
CI	2.4	2.4
PA	40/23	35/20
PCWP	22	17
CVP	12	9

(A) yes, based on the reduced pulmonary capillary wedge pressure and increased stroke index
(B) no, since the cardiac index did not improve
(C) no, based on the decrease in blood pressure
(D) yes, based on the stable cardiac index

Questions 148 and 149 refer to the following scenario.

A 45-year-old male is admitted to your unit with the diagnosis of status asthmaticus. He requires intubation and is placed on mechanical ventilation in the AMV (assist/control) mode with a tidal volume of 850 cc and a respiratory rate of 10. He is, however, very anxious and is triggering the ventilator at a rate of 40 bpm. His FIO_2 is 0.40 and no PEEP (positive end expiratory pressure) is present. He has the following set of blood gas values at this time:

pH	7.34
PaCO$_2$	30
PaO$_2$	54
HCO$_3^-$	18

He is attempting to pull the endotracheal tube out due to anxiety or confusion. The physician requests the administration of 10 mg of Versed to manage the anxiety. After administering the sedative, his respiratory rate changes from 40 to 10. His pulse oximeter now reads 0.95.

148. At this point, what should be done to monitor his status?

(A) obtain a set of arterial blood gas values

(B) continue monitoring his SpO$_2$ values

(C) obtain a set of electrolyte values to search for the cause of the metabolic acidosis

(D) No further assessment is necessary at this point since the respiratory rate has fallen to desirable levels.

149. With the administration of the Versed, the respiratory rate decreased from 40 to 10. What is the possible effect of this change in respiratory rate?

(A) development of a metabolic acidosis

(B) development of a respiratory acidosis

(C) No major effect will occur as long as the SpO$_2$ is normal.

(D) No major effect will occur as long as the ventilator rate is maintained at least at 10.

150. Which of the following are considered to be effective preload-reducing agents in the presence of acute left ventricular failure?

I. furosemide (Lasix)

II. nitroprusside

III. nitroglycerine

(A) I and II

(B) I and III

(C) II and III

(D) I, II, and III

151. A 34-year-old female has been in your unit for two days for coma of unknown origin. She was admitted from her home, with her family stating that she has been "sick for a few days." Upon admission, she was unresponsive and required intubation in the emergency room. She presently has a Glasgow Coma Score of 3. Her pupils are fixed and unresponsive. Her body temperature is 38°C. She currently is on a ventilator in the AMV (assist/control) mode, with a ventilator rate of 12 and a total rate of 15. The physician wants to obtain an EEG to help establish brain death. Based on the preceding information, do arguments exist to support obtaining an EEG?

(A) Yes, it will provide definitive evidence of brain death.
(B) Yes, although it will not alone support brain death, it will confirm brain death in the presence of a Glasgow Coma Score of 3.
(C) No, since the patient is breathing spontaneously brain death cannot be present.
(D) No, since not enough time has passed to attempt to establish brain death.

152. Assume that you have a patient with the following hemodynamic information:

blood pressure	124/74
pulse	109
CI	1.8
PA	33/20
PCWP	17
CVP	12

Give an example of a medication combination that would be most effective in treating these hemodynamics.

   I. dobutamine
  II. captopril
 III. Lasix

    (A) I and II
    (B) I and III
    (C) II and III
    (D) I, II, and III

Questions 153 and 154 refer to the following scenario.

A 71-year-old male is admitted to your unit following an exacerbation of COPD (chronic obstructive pulmonary disease). He currently is short of breath but is not orthopneic. He has generalized expiratory wheezing and diffuse crackles. He appears to be slightly malnourished and underweight. He is on oxygen at 0.40 via a Venti-mask. His admission blood gases reveal the following information:

pH	7.34
PaCO$_2$	42
PaO$_2$	87
HCO$_3^-$	26

153. The physician states that he has a large intrapulmonary shunt. If you wanted to estimate this patient's intrapulmonary shunt, measurement of which parameters would allow this estimate?

   I. A-a (alveolar-arterial) gradient
   II. a/A (arterial/alveolar) ratio
   III. PaO$_2$/FIO$_2$ ratio

   (A) I and II
   (B) I and III
   (C) II and III
   (D) I, II, and III

154. Which form of COPD (chronic obstructive pulmonary disease) is likely to predominate in this patient?

   (A) chronic bronchitis
   (B) asthma
   (C) emphysema
   (D) bronchiectasis

155. Following repair of an abdominal aortic aneurysm, a 55-year-old male is admitted to your unit for postoperative management. Which of the following would be factors to consider as potential complications following this type of surgery?

   I. decreased urine output
   II. loss of pedal pulses
   III. cyanosis of the feet

   (A) I and II
   (B) I and III
   (C) II and III
   (D) I, II, and III

156. A 55-year-old male in your unit has been diagnosed as septic secondary to a hepatic abscess. The physician has requested that a fluid bolus of normal saline be given to support his hemodynamics. What is the rationale for this therapy?

   (A) to offset the loss of preload secondary to vasodilation
   (B) to increase afterload secondary to vasodilation
   (C) to raise the capillary osmotic pressure
   (D) to compensate for the reduction in hemoglobin carrying capacity

157. In sepsis, one substrate that is normally not used for energy becomes preferentially catabolized. What is this substrate?

(A) fat
(B) carbohydrate
(C) phospholipid
(D) protein

158. A 31-year-old female with a history of mental retardation is admitted to your unit following a respiratory arrest. She has a parasympathetic disorder that causes excessive parasympathetic tone. What will be the primary pulmonary effect of the increased parasympathetic tone?

 I. decreased pulmonary macrophage activity
 II. increased bronchial secretions
III. excessive airway reactivity

(A) I and III
(B) II and III
(C) I
(D) II

159. Increased secretions and mucous plugging will potentially result in which clinical condition?

(A) CHF (congestive heart failure)
(B) atelectasis
(C) increased physiologic dead space
(D) chronic lung disease

Questions 160 and 161 refer to the following scenario.

A 56-year-old male is in your unit following an episode of shortness of breath. Upon physical examination, he is short of breath, has 3+ pitting edema of both lower legs, and has generalized crackles throughout both lung fields. His vital signs are as follows:

blood pressure	136/82
pulse	113
respiratory rate	36
temperature	37.7°C

A pulmonary artery catheter reveals the following information:

CI	2.7
PA	56/38
PCWP	14
CVP	18

160. Based on these symptoms, which condition is likely to be present?

   (A) right ventricular failure
   (B) left ventricular failure
   (C) biventricular failure
   (D) sepsis-induced respiratory failure

161. Which therapy would most likely help improve these symptoms?

   I. oxygen therapy
   II. Lasix
   III. prostaglandin E_1
      (A) I and II
      (B) I and III
      (C) II and III
      (D) I, II, and III

Questions 162 and 163 refer to the following scenario.

A 64-year-old male is admitted to your unit with shortness of breath. He has never before been to a physician, stating that "I've never been sick." He states that he has smoked about one pack of unfiltered cigarettes a day since he was a teenager. He has marked inspiratory wheezing with scattered coarse crackles. He is coughing large amounts of yellowish-green sputum and states that he normally coughs, mostly in the morning. The change in color of the sputum from white to the present color has occurred within the past two days. His blood gases reveals the following information:

pH	7.35
$PaCO_2$	48
PaO_2	57
HCO_3^-	25

162. Based on the preceding information, which condition is likely to be present?

   I. reactive airway disease
   II. small (oat) cell cancer
   III. pneumonia
      (A) I and II
      (B) I and III
      (C) II and III
      (D) I, II, and III

163. Which therapies are most likely to help improve his symptoms immediately?

    I. parasympathetic stimulators
    II. theophylline
    III. beta stimulants

      (A) I and II
      (B) I and III
      (C) II and III
      (D) I, II, and III

164. When the pH falls with a metabolic acidosis, what is the response of other electrolytes?

    I. potassium increases
    II. sodium falls
    III. bicarbonate decreases

      (A) I and II
      (B) I and III
      (C) II and III
      (D) I, II, and III

Questions 165 and 166 refer to the following scenario.

Following a code, a 77-year-old female is admitted to your unit for management. She is awake and alert but states that her chest is "sore." During your shift, you note that her blood pressure decreases from 118/78 to 98/66 during spontaneous breathing. Upon auscultation, her heart sounds are muffled and distant, although S_1 and S_2 are audible. She does not indicate that any discomfort exists. A 12-lead ECG is free of any injury pattern, although the voltage (ECG height) is diminished.

165. Based on the preceding information, what condition is likely to be developing?

    (A) pericardial tamponade
    (B) CHF (congestive heart failure)
    (C) pericarditis
    (D) Prinzmetal's angina

166. What is the most effective treatment for this condition?

    (A) pericardiocentesis
    (B) aspirin
    (C) beta blockade
    (D) nitroglycerine

167. A 44-year-old female is in your unit following a pulmonary resection of her left lower lobe due to primary large cell cancer. She is recovering uneventfully, although on the third postoperative day she is still intubated. Following a series of coughs, she indicates that she feels short of breath and is becoming anxious. When you listen to her you notice a sound like air rushing out of the back of her throat. The low-pressure and low-volume alarm on the ventilator now activate. Based on this information, what is likely to be occurring?

(A) pneumothorax
(B) tracheal tear
(C) mispositioning of the endotracheal tube
(D) tearing of the balloon on the endotracheal tube

168. Which of the following is considered most helpful in determining the presence or absence of brain death?

(A) EEG (electroencephalogram)
(B) MRI (magnetic resonance imaging)
(C) skull x-rays
(D) cerebral angiography

169. A 49-year-old male is in your unit following a two-story fall from an apartment window. He has a fractured skull, is unresponsive, and has equal but dilated, unresponsive pupils. The physician wants to reduce the ICP (intracranial pressure) rapidly, based on the potential for elevation of the ICP. Which of the following therapies would be effective in reducing the ICP rapidly?

I. hyperoxygenation
II. hyperventilation
III. use of an osmotic diuretic (e.g., mannitol)

    (A) I and II
    (B) I and III
    (C) II and III
    (D) I, II, and III

Questions 170 and 171 refer to the following scenario.

A 49-year-old male is admitted to your unit with persistent chest pain. He complains of chest pain that is unrelieved by rest, although the pain worsens upon inspiration. He states that the pain has been present for about 24 hours. His ECG demonstrates ST elevation in leads I, II, and III, aVL, aVF, and V_1 to V_5. Auscultation of the heart and lungs reveals no overt abnormalities.

170. Based on the preceding information, which condition is likely to be developing?

(A) anterior/lateral MI (myocardial infarction)
(B) inferior/anterior MI
(C) pericardial tamponade
(D) pericarditis

171. What would be the most effective treatment in this situation?

(A) thrombolytics
(B) afterload reduction
(C) steroids
(D) analgesics

172. Interpret the following 12-lead ECG.

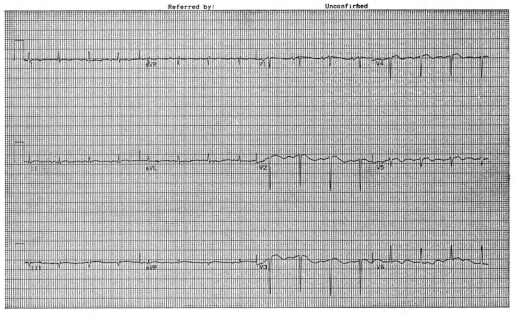

(A) inferior MI (myocardial infarction)
(B) anterior MI
(C) lateral ischemia
(D) subendocardial MI

173. A 49-year-old male in your unit with cirrhosis is slightly hypotensive (blood pressure 96/58) and tachycardic (113). He has marked ascites, which results in his "sort of having a hard time breathing." Based on this information, what would most likely be done to improve his comfort level?

(A) pericentesis
(B) use of a semi-Fowler's position
(C) administration of 25 g of intravenous albumin
(D) peritoneal dialysis

174. A 28-year-old female is admitted to your unit with the diagnosis of supra-ventricular paroxsymal tachycardia. Physical measures to slow the heart rate have failed. The physician elects to try a rapid-acting pharmacologic therapy in an attempt to break the tachycardia. Which of the following could be utilized for this therapy?

    I. esmolol
    II. verapamil
    III. adenosine
        (A) I and II
        (B) I and III
        (C) II and III
        (D) I, II, and III

175. A 51-year-old male is admitted to your unit following a pancreatectomy. Which of the following therapies will need to be administered to replace the loss of pancreatic function?

    I. insulin
    II. trypsin
    III. exogenous bilirubin
        (A) I and II
        (B) I and III
        (C) II and III
        (D) I, II, and III

176. A 76-year-old female is admitted to your unit with the chief complaint of nausea, vomiting, and cramping pain in the epigastric region. Her abdomen is distended and is hyperresonant upon percussion. Bowel sounds are distant. Based on this information, which condition is likely to be developing?

    (A) perforation of the small intestine
    (B) obstruction of the small intestine
    (C) pancreatitis
    (D) obstruction of the large intestine

177. Which of the following are characteristic of left bundle branch block?

   I. Qs in V_1
   II. Rs wave in II, III, and aVF
   III. Wide, notched QRS in V_5 and V_6

   (A) I and II
   (B) I and III
   (C) II and III
   (D) I, II, and III

178. A 66-year-old male is in your unit following a CABG (coronary artery bypass graft). Postoperatively his recovery has been complicated by a low urine output and fluid retention. He is to be started on continuous arterial venous hemodialysis. Which of the following will be effectively treated by this therapy?

   I. fluid removal
   II. elimination of potassium
   III. elimination of creatinine

   (A) I and II
   (B) I and III
   (C) II and III
   (D) I, II, and III

179. Loss of R-wave progression in the precordial leads might indicate which of the following?

   (A) LV hypertrophy
   (B) RV atrophy
   (C) pericardial tamponade and pericarditis
   (D) loss of ventricular muscle mass

180. During the measurement of a patient's cardiac output, you note that the cardiac output values flucutate as follows:

first measurement	5.1
second measurement	3.3
third measurement	3.7
fourth measurement	4.8

The average cardiac output based upon these readings is 3.93 LPM. A new nurse asks if the variation seen in the above readings is normal. When explaining ·the variations, which of the following would be considered accurate statements regarding the thermodilution cardiac output technique.

I. All values should be within 10% of each other.
II. The first reading is frequently inaccurate.
III. The Fick equation is used to check the acccuracy of the thermodilution cardiac output.

    (A) I and II
    (B) I and III
    (C) II and III
    (D) I, II, and III

181. Right ventricular hypertrophy is characterized by which of the following?

    I. large Q waves in I and aVL
   II. larger R wave than S wave in V_1
  III. large R wave in V_{3R}

    (A) I and II
    (B) I and III
    (C) II and III
    (D) I, II, and III

182. A 79-year-old female is admitted from a nursing home with the diagnosis of hypotension. The following clinical and laboratory data are available:

blood pressure	88/50
pulse	116
respiratory rate	30
temperature	38
SpO_2	0.94
Na^+	156
K^+	4.7
Cl^-	120
HCO_3^-	21
albumin	3.6
urinary Na^+	33
urinary osmolality	643

Her lung sounds are clear, her heart sounds fast but normal, and she has dark, concentrated urine. Based on this information, which condition is likely to be developing?

    (A) acute renal failure
    (B) dehydration
    (C) left ventricular failure
    (D) acute nutritional failure

183. Which therapy would most likely help this condition?

    (A) fluid bolus of 500 cc D_5W
    (B) Na^+ restriction
    (C) dobutamine
    (D) hyperalimentation

Questions 184 and 185 refer to the following scenario.

A 76-year-old male is admitted from the emergency room complaining of persistent, although intermittent, chest pain. His pain started on Friday (three days ago) and has been intermittent since that time. The pain is severe at times and is unrelieved by rest or position changes. He did not want to come to the hospital since he did not want to bother his physician over the weekend. His admission ECG shows a large R wave in V_1 and V_2 with 2-mm ST depression in II, III, and aVF.

184. Based on the preceding information, which condition is likely to be present?

    (A) anterior MI (myocardial infarction)
    (B) posterior MI
    (C) inferior ischemia
    (D) pericarditis

185. Which cardiac isoenzymes might be useful in identifying whether an MI has occurred?

    (A) CPK-MB of 5% of total CPK
    (B) CPK-MM > CPK MB
    (C) LDH-1 > LDH-2
    (D) CPK total of 80

186. Which of the following would be indications for initiating ICP (intracranial pressure) monitoring?

    I. closed head injury
    II. cerebellar infarction
    III. postoperative craniotomy management
        (A) I and II
        (B) I and III
        (C) II and III
        (D) I, II, and III

187. Which of the following statements regarding thrombolytic therapy is true?

(A) Tissue plasminogen activators are the most reliable thrombolytic in lysing coronary thrombi.

(B) Streptokinase is the most reliable thrombolytic in lysing coronary thrombi.

(C) Aspirin and heparin can effectively lyse most coronary thrombi.

(D) No thrombolytic has yet demonstrated superiority in clot lysing.

Questions 188 and 189 refer to the following scenario.

A 47-year-old male is admitted to your unit following a house fire. He made repeated efforts to enter his house to evacuate his three children, who were trapped in the house. He was rescued by fire department personnel after he had collapsed in the house. He now is admitted with second-degree burns over 30% of his body, primarily involving his arms, face, and back. He is awake but in considerable pain. He does not complain of any shortness of breath and his pulse oximeter registers a value of 100.

188. Based on the preceding information, which laboratory data would be useful?

(A) coagulation profile
(B) urine electrolyte values to rule out rhabdomyolysis
(C) serum albumin levels
(D) carboxyhemoglobin levels

189. Which of the following therapies will most likely be employed to help treat the burn wounds?

I. silver maleate ointment
II. Neosporin ointment
III. silver sulfadiazine ointment

(A) I and II
(B) I and III
(C) II and III
(D) I, II, and III

190. A 67-year-old female is admitted to your unit with atrial fibrillation. On her echocardiogram, she is noted to have a large mural thrombus. Of the following conditions, which would NOT be potential complications of this atrial thrombus?

(A) pulmonary emboli
(B) CVA (cerebrovascular accident)
(C) loss of pulse in either hand
(D) loss of pulse in lower legs

191. Interpret the following ECG rhythm strip:

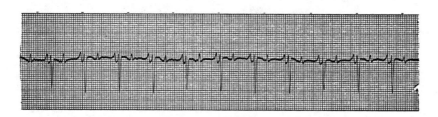

    (A) atrial flutter with block
    (B) atrial tachycardia with block
    (C) atrial fibrillation
    (D) second-degree type 2 heart block

Questions 192 and 193 refer to the following scenario.

A 71-year-old male is in your unit following a CABG (coronary artery bypass graft). His inital postoperative recovery is uneventful and he is extubated eight hours after returning to the unit. At 0400, you note that his mediastinal chest tube has drained 200 cc in the past hour. He has the following hemodynamics at 0400:

blood pressure	102/70
pulse	88
CI	2.5
PA	26/12
PCWP	11
CVP	5

His lung sounds are clear and he does not complain of any change in his discomfort level.

192. Based on the preceding situation, which condition is likely to be present?

    (A) normal postoperative mediastinal drainage
    (B) mediastinal bleeding, indicating that major postoperative bleeding is present
    (C) developing hemothorax
    (D) cardiac tamponade

193. If the condition were clinically significant, which clinical indicators would be present?

    I. orthopnea
    II. decreased stroke volume/index
    III. decreased PCWP (pulmonary capillary wedge pressure)

(A) I and II
(B) I and III
(C) II and III
(D) I, II, and III

Questions 194 and 195 refer to the following scenario.

A 34-year-old female is admitted to your unit with the diagnosis of possible pulmonary embolism. She complains of shortness of breath and inspiratory right side chest pain. Her respiratory rate is 34 and minute ventilation is 14 LPM. Analysis of her blood gases reveals the following:

pH	7.52
$PaCO_2$	25
PaO_2	68
HCO_3^-	24
FIO_2	0.28

194. Based on the preceding information, which of the above are consistent with the diagnosis of pulmonary emboli?

   I. minute ventilation of 14 LPM
   II. PaO_2 of 68 on 28% oxygen
   III. HCO_3^- of 24

   (A) I and II
   (B) I and III
   (C) II and III
   (D) I, II, and III

195. If a pulmonary embolism is present, what happens to the physiologic dead space of the lung?

   (A) remains normal
   (B) increases
   (C) decreases
   (D) initally elevates, then falls

196. In cardiac tamponade, which of the following clinical indicators may be present?

   I. equalization of CVP (central venous pressure) and PCWP (pulmonary capillary wedge pressure)
   II. reduced stroke volume/index
   III. pulsus paradoxus

   (A) I and II
   (B) I and III
   (C) II and III
   (D) I, II, and III

197. A 54-year-old male is to be transferred from your unit pending analysis of his morning blood gas values. He was initially admitted to the unit with the diagnosis of COPD (chronic obstructive pulmonary disease) with an acute exacerbation. He currently is alert and oriented, although he has mild shortness of breath and has peripheral cyanosis and "clubbing" of his fingernails. His blood gas values are as follows:

pH	7.35
$PaCO_2$	89
PaO_2	62
HCO_3^-	41

Based on the preceding information, what should be done?

(A) consider intubation and mechanical ventilation
(B) initiate high-flow oxygen therapy and discharge the patient from the unit
(C) keep the patient in the unit and start nasal CPAP (continuous positive airway pressure)
(D) proceed with discharge from the unit

198. When administering an angiotension converting enzyme inhibitor (such as captopril or enalapril), which of the following would be monitored to assess the effectiveness of the therapy?

(A) PCWP (pulmonary capillary wedge pressure)
(B) CVP (central venous pressure)
(C) heart rate
(D) SVR (systemic vascular resistance)

Questions 199 and 200 refer to the following scenario.

A 66-year-old male is admitted to your unit with the diagnosis of acute anginal episode. He currently has the following vital signs:

blood pressure	168/104
pulse	82
respiratory rate	28
temperature	37.3°C

His skin is cool and he is diaphoretic. He currently denies having any chest pain.

199. In order to reduce his chest pain effectively, which of the following therapies may be utililzed?

   I. nitroglycerine
  II. nitroprusside
 III. dobutamine

    (A) I and II
    (B) I and III
    (C) II and III
    (D) I, II, and III

200. What is the likely precipitating mechanism for the anginal episode?

    (A) increased myocardial oxygen consumption
    (B) reduced left ventricular stroke work index
    (C) increased end diastolic and wedge pressures
    (D) increased systemic oxygen consumption

CONGRATULATIONS!

You have finished the exam. Review it to cover any problematic questions. Do
not change any answers unless you are sure the change is necessary. Compare
your results with the answers beginning on p. 348. Do not immediately grade
your test. After reviewing the exam, take some time to relax before returning to
grade your test and study any areas you missed. Note the areas in which you
need improvement. This test is an approximation of the actual CCRN exam and
should give you a rough idea of how you will do on the exam. Reread in the text
any areas in which your success rate was less than 70%. We wish you luck in
the actual exam. You are to be congratulated for taking the time and effort to
prepare for it.

PART II

Answer Sheets
for Practice
Exams

CHAPTER 1 —————————————

Cardiovascular Practice Exam

1. ———	32. ———	63. ———	94. ———
2. ———	33. ———	64. ———	95. ———
3. ———	34. ———	65. ———	96. ———
4. ———	35. ———	66. ———	97. ———
5. ———	36. ———	67. ———	98. ———
6. ———	37. ———	68. ———	99. ———
7. ———	38. ———	69. ———	100. ———
8. ———	39. ———	70. ———	101. ———
9. ———	40. ———	71. ———	102. ———
10. ———	41. ———	72. ———	103. ———
11. ———	42. ———	73. ———	104. ———
12. ———	43. ———	74. ———	105. ———
13. ———	44. ———	75. ———	106. ———
14. ———	45. ———	76. ———	107. ———
15. ———	46. ———	77. ———	108. ———
16. ———	47. ———	78. ———	109. ———
17. ———	48. ———	79. ———	110. ———
18. ———	49. ———	80. ———	111. ———
19. ———	50. ———	81. ———	112. ———
20. ———	51. ———	82. ———	113. ———
21. ———	52. ———	83. ———	114. ———
22. ———	53. ———	84. ———	115. ———
23. ———	54. ———	85. ———	116. ———
24. ———	55. ———	86. ———	117. ———
25. ———	56. ———	87. ———	118. ———
26. ———	57. ———	88. ———	119. ———
27. ———	58. ———	89. ———	120. ———
28. ———	59. ———	90. ———	121. ———
29. ———	60. ———	91. ———	122. ———
30. ———	61. ———	92. ———	123. ———
31. ———	62. ———	93. ———	124. ———

125. _____
126. _____
127. _____
128. _____
129. _____
130. _____
131. _____
132. _____
133. _____
134. _____
135. _____
136. _____
137. _____
138. _____
139. _____
140. _____
141. _____

142. _____
143. _____
144. _____
145. _____
146. _____
147. _____
148. _____
149. _____
150. _____
151. _____
152. _____
153. _____
154. _____
155. _____
156. _____
157. _____

158. _____
159. _____
160. _____
161. _____
162. _____
163. _____
164. _____
165. _____
166. _____
167. _____
168. _____
169. _____
170. _____
171. _____
172. _____
173. _____

174. _____
175. _____
176. _____
177. _____
178. _____
179. _____
180. _____
181. _____
182. _____
183. _____
184. _____
185. _____
186. _____
187. _____
188. _____
189. _____

CHAPTER 2 ──────────────────────

Pulmonary Practice Exam

1. ────	32. ────	63. ────	94. ────
2. ────	33. ────	64. ────	95. ────
3. ────	34. ────	65. ────	96. ────
4. ────	35. ────	66. ────	97. ────
5. ────	36. ────	67. ────	98. ────
6. ────	37. ────	68. ────	99. ────
7. ────	38. ────	69. ────	100. ────
8. ────	39. ────	70. ────	101. ────
9. ────	40. ────	71. ────	102. ────
10. ────	41. ────	72. ────	103. ────
11. ────	42. ────	73. ────	104. ────
12. ────	43. ────	74. ────	105. ────
13. ────	44. ────	75. ────	106. ────
14. ────	45. ────	76. ────	107. ────
15. ────	46. ────	77. ────	108. ────
16. ────	47. ────	78. ────	109. ────
17. ────	48. ────	79. ────	110. ────
18. ────	49. ────	80. ────	111. ────
19. ────	50. ────	81. ────	112. ────
20. ────	51. ────	82. ────	113. ────
21. ────	52. ────	83. ────	114. ────
22. ────	53. ────	84. ────	115. ────
23. ────	54. ────	85. ────	116. ────
24. ────	55. ────	86. ────	117. ────
25. ────	56. ────	87. ────	118. ────
26. ────	57. ────	88. ────	119. ────
27. ────	58. ────	89. ────	120. ────
28. ────	59. ────	90. ────	121. ────
29. ────	60. ────	91. ────	122. ────
30. ────	61. ────	92. ────	123. ────
31. ────	62. ────	93. ────	124. ────

125. _____   128. _____   131. _____   133. _____
126. _____   129. _____   132. _____   134. _____
127. _____   130. _____

CHAPTER 3 —————————————————

Neurology Practice Exam

1. ———	32. ———	63. ———	94. ———
2. ———	33. ———	64. ———	95. ———
3. ———	34. ———	65. ———	96. ———
4. ———	35. ———	66. ———	97. ———
5. ———	36. ———	67. ———	98. ———
6. ———	37. ———	68. ———	99. ———
7. ———	38. ———	69. ———	100. ———
8. ———	39. ———	70. ———	101. ———
9. ———	40. ———	71. ———	102. ———
10. ———	41. ———	72. ———	103. ———
11. ———	42. ———	73. ———	104. ———
12. ———	43. ———	74. ———	105. ———
13. ———	44. ———	75. ———	106. ———
14. ———	45. ———	76. ———	107. ———
15. ———	46. ———	77. ———	108. ———
16. ———	47. ———	78. ———	109. ———
17. ———	48. ———	79. ———	110. ———
18. ———	49. ———	80. ———	111. ———
19. ———	50. ———	81. ———	112. ———
20. ———	51. ———	82. ———	113. ———
21. ———	52. ———	83. ———	114. ———
22. ———	53. ———	84. ———	115. ———
23. ———	54. ———	85. ———	116. ———
24. ———	55. ———	86. ———	117. ———
25. ———	56. ———	87. ———	118. ———
26. ———	57. ———	88. ———	119. ———
27. ———	58. ———	89. ———	120. ———
28. ———	59. ———	90. ———	121. ———
29. ———	60. ———	91. ———	122. ———
30. ———	61. ———	92. ———	123. ———
31. ———	62. ———	93. ———	124. ———

125. ———
126. ———
127. ———
128. ———
129. ———
130. ———
131. ———

132. ———
133. ———
134. ———
135. ———
136. ———
137. ———
138. ———

139. ———
140. ———
141. ———
142. ———
143. ———
144. ———

145. ———
146. ———
147. ———
148. ———
149. ———
150. ———

CHAPTER 4 _____

Gastroenterology Practice Exam

1. _____	21. _____	41. _____	60. _____
2. _____	22. _____	42. _____	61. _____
3. _____	23. _____	43. _____	62. _____
4. _____	24. _____	44. _____	63. _____
5. _____	25. _____	45. _____	64. _____
6. _____	26. _____	46. _____	65. _____
7. _____	27. _____	47. _____	66. _____
8. _____	28. _____	48. _____	67. _____
9. _____	29. _____	49. _____	68. _____
10. _____	30. _____	50. _____	69. _____
11. _____	31. _____	51. _____	70. _____
12. _____	32. _____	52. _____	71. _____
13. _____	33. _____	53. _____	72. _____
14. _____	34. _____	54. _____	73. _____
15. _____	35. _____	55. _____	74. _____
16. _____	36. _____	56. _____	75. _____
17. _____	37. _____	57. _____	76. _____
18. _____	38. _____	58. _____	77. _____
19. _____	39. _____	59. _____	78. _____
20. _____	40. _____		

CHAPTER 5 _____

Renal Practice Exam

1. _____	20. _____	39. _____	58. _____
2. _____	21. _____	40. _____	59. _____
3. _____	22. _____	41. _____	60. _____
4. _____	23. _____	42. _____	61. _____
5. _____	24. _____	43. _____	62. _____
6. _____	25. _____	44. _____	63. _____
7. _____	26. _____	45. _____	64. _____
8. _____	27. _____	46. _____	65. _____
9. _____	28. _____	47. _____	66. _____
10. _____	29. _____	48. _____	67. _____
11. _____	30. _____	49. _____	68. _____
12. _____	31. _____	50. _____	69. _____
13. _____	32. _____	51. _____	70. _____
14. _____	33. _____	52. _____	71. _____
15. _____	34. _____	53. _____	72. _____
16. _____	35. _____	54. _____	73. _____
17. _____	36. _____	55. _____	74. _____
18. _____	37. _____	56. _____	75. _____
19. _____	38. _____	57. _____	

CHAPTER 6 ——————————————————————

Endocrine Practice Exam

1. ——————
2. ——————
3. ——————
4. ——————
5. ——————
6. ——————
7. ——————
8. ——————
9. ——————
10. ——————
11. ——————
12. ——————
13. ——————
14. ——————
15. ——————
16. ——————

17. ——————
18. ——————
19. ——————
20. ——————
21. ——————
22. ——————
23. ——————
24. ——————
25. ——————
26. ——————
27. ——————
28. ——————
29. ——————
30. ——————
31. ——————
32. ——————

33. ——————
34. ——————
35. ——————
36. ——————
37. ——————
38. ——————
39. ——————
40. ——————
41. ——————
42. ——————
43. ——————
44. ——————
45. ——————
46. ——————
47. ——————

48. ——————
49. ——————
50. ——————
51. ——————
52. ——————
53. ——————
54. ——————
55. ——————
56. ——————
57. ——————
58. ——————
59. ——————
60. ——————
61. ——————
62. ——————

CHAPTER 7

Immunology and Hematology Practice Exam

1. _____	17. _____	33. _____	48. _____
2. _____	18. _____	34. _____	49. _____
3. _____	19. _____	35. _____	50. _____
4. _____	20. _____	36. _____	51. _____
5. _____	21. _____	37. _____	52. _____
6. _____	22. _____	38. _____	53. _____
7. _____	23. _____	39. _____	54. _____
8. _____	24. _____	40. _____	55. _____
9. _____	25. _____	41. _____	56. _____
10. _____	26. _____	42. _____	57. _____
11. _____	27. _____	43. _____	58. _____
12. _____	28. _____	44. _____	59. _____
13. _____	29. _____	45. _____	60. _____
14. _____	30. _____	46. _____	61. _____
15. _____	31. _____	47. _____	62. _____
16. _____	32. _____		

CHAPTER 8

Multisystem Organ Dysfunction Practice Exam

1. _____	12. _____	23. _____	34. _____
2. _____	13. _____	24. _____	35. _____
3. _____	14. _____	25. _____	36. _____
4. _____	15. _____	26. _____	37. _____
5. _____	16. _____	27. _____	38. _____
6. _____	17. _____	28. _____	39. _____
7. _____	18. _____	29. _____	40. _____
8. _____	19. _____	30. _____	41. _____
9. _____	20. _____	31. _____	42. _____
10. _____	21. _____	32. _____	43. _____
11. _____	22. _____	33. _____	44. _____

CHAPTER 9 _____

Comprehensive Practice Exam—1

1. _____	30. _____	59. _____	88. _____
2. _____	31. _____	60. _____	89. _____
3. _____	32. _____	61. _____	90. _____
4. _____	33. _____	62. _____	91. _____
5. _____	34. _____	63. _____	92. _____
6. _____	35. _____	64. _____	93. _____
7. _____	36. _____	65. _____	94. _____
8. _____	37. _____	66. _____	95. _____
9. _____	38. _____	67. _____	96. _____
10. _____	39. _____	68. _____	97. _____
11. _____	40. _____	69. _____	98. _____
12. _____	41. _____	70. _____	99. _____
13. _____	42. _____	71. _____	100. _____
14. _____	43. _____	72. _____	101. _____
15. _____	44. _____	73. _____	102. _____
16. _____	45. _____	74. _____	103. _____
17. _____	46. _____	75. _____	104. _____
18. _____	47. _____	76. _____	105. _____
19. _____	48. _____	77. _____	106. _____
20. _____	49. _____	78. _____	107. _____
21. _____	50. _____	79. _____	108. _____
22. _____	51. _____	80. _____	109. _____
23. _____	52. _____	81. _____	110. _____
24. _____	53. _____	82. _____	111. _____
25. _____	54. _____	83. _____	112. _____
26. _____	55. _____	84. _____	113. _____
27. _____	56. _____	85. _____	114. _____
28. _____	57. _____	86. _____	115. _____
29. _____	58. _____	87. _____	116. _____

117. _____	138. _____	159. _____	180. _____
118. _____	139. _____	160. _____	181. _____
119. _____	140. _____	161. _____	182. _____
120. _____	141. _____	162. _____	183. _____
121. _____	142. _____	163. _____	184. _____
122. _____	143. _____	164. _____	185. _____
123. _____	144. _____	165. _____	186. _____
124. _____	145. _____	166. _____	187. _____
125. _____	146. _____	167. _____	188. _____
126. _____	147. _____	168. _____	189. _____
127. _____	148. _____	169. _____	190. _____
128. _____	149. _____	170. _____	191. _____
129. _____	150. _____	171. _____	192. _____
130. _____	151. _____	172. _____	193. _____
131. _____	152. _____	173. _____	194. _____
132. _____	153. _____	174. _____	195. _____
133. _____	154. _____	175. _____	196. _____
134. _____	155. _____	176. _____	197. _____
135. _____	156. _____	177. _____	198. _____
136. _____	157. _____	178. _____	199. _____
137. _____	158. _____	179. _____	200. _____

CHAPTER 10 _____

Comprehensive Practice Exam—2

1. _____	30. _____	59. _____	88. _____
2. _____	31. _____	60. _____	89. _____
3. _____	32. _____	61. _____	90. _____
4. _____	33. _____	62. _____	91. _____
5. _____	34. _____	63. _____	92. _____
6. _____	35. _____	64. _____	93. _____
7. _____	36. _____	65. _____	94. _____
8. _____	37. _____	66. _____	95. _____
9. _____	38. _____	67. _____	96. _____
10. _____	39. _____	68. _____	97. _____
11. _____	40. _____	69. _____	98. _____
12. _____	41. _____	70. _____	99. _____
13. _____	42. _____	71. _____	100. _____
14. _____	43. _____	72. _____	101. _____
15. _____	44. _____	73. _____	102. _____
16. _____	45. _____	74. _____	103. _____
17. _____	46. _____	75. _____	104. _____
18. _____	47. _____	76. _____	105. _____
19. _____	48. _____	77. _____	106. _____
20. _____	49. _____	78. _____	107. _____
21. _____	50. _____	79. _____	108. _____
22. _____	51. _____	80. _____	109. _____
23. _____	52. _____	81. _____	110. _____
24. _____	53. _____	82. _____	111. _____
25. _____	54. _____	83. _____	112. _____
26. _____	55. _____	84. _____	113. _____
27. _____	56. _____	85. _____	114. _____
28. _____	57. _____	86. _____	115. _____
29. _____	58. _____	87. _____	116. _____

117. _____	138. _____	159. _____	180. _____
118. _____	139. _____	160. _____	181. _____
119. _____	140. _____	161. _____	182. _____
120. _____	141. _____	162. _____	183. _____
121. _____	142. _____	163. _____	184. _____
122. _____	143. _____	164. _____	185. _____
123. _____	144. _____	165. _____	186. _____
124. _____	145. _____	166. _____	187. _____
125. _____	146. _____	167. _____	188. _____
126. _____	147. _____	168. _____	189. _____
127. _____	148. _____	169. _____	190. _____
128. _____	149. _____	170. _____	191. _____
129. _____	150. _____	171. _____	192. _____
130. _____	151. _____	172. _____	193. _____
131. _____	152. _____	173. _____	194. _____
132. _____	153. _____	174. _____	195. _____
133. _____	154. _____	175. _____	196. _____
134. _____	155. _____	176. _____	197. _____
135. _____	156. _____	177. _____	198. _____
136. _____	157. _____	178. _____	199. _____
137. _____	158. _____	179. _____	200. _____

PART III

Answers to Practice Exams

CHAPTER 1 ────────────────────

Cardiovascular Practice Exam

1. _A_*p 16*
2. _D_*p 11*
3. _A_*p 11*
4. _D_*p 11*
5. _C_*p 17*
6. _A_*p 17*
7. _D_*p 4*
8. _C_*p 14*
9. _B_*p 16*
10. _D_*p 16*
11. _A_*p 10*
12. _B_*p 20*
13. _D_*p 20*
14. _A_*p 17*
15. _B_*p 17*
16. _D_*p 17*
17. _A_*p 20*
18. _A_*p 17*
19. _A_*p 11–12*
20. _D_*p 11*
21. _A_*p 16*
22. _B_*p 12, 87*
23. _A_*p 16*
24. _A_*p 17*
25. _B_*p 10*
26. _A_*p 10*
27. _D_*p 20*
28. _A_*p 8*
29. _D_*p 8*
30. _A_*p 8*
31. _D_*p 8*

32. _B_*p 8*
33. _A_*p 9*
34. _A_*p 12*
35. _C_*p 15*
36. _D_*p 16*
37. _D_*p 16*
38. _C_*p 17*
39. _A_*p 16–17*
40. _A_*p 18*
41. _B_*p 19*
42. _C_*p 20*
43. _D_*p 48*
44. _D_*p 54*
45. _D_*p 48*
46. _A_*p 48*
47. _B_*p 48*
48. _D_*p 65*
49. _C_*p 53*
50. _B_*p 53*
51. _A_*p 33*
52. _B_*p 35*
53. _D_*p 38*
54. _C_*p 38*
55. _D_*p 46–47*
56. _A_*p 43*
57. _C_*p 45*
58. _B_*p 44*
59. _B_*p 53*
60. _A_*p 52*
61. _C_*p 55*
62. _B_*p 53*

63. _B_*p 53*
64. _A_*p 65*
65. _A_*p 50*
66. _B_*p 50*
67. _C_*p 48*
68. _D_*p 48*
69. _C_*p 43*
70. _D_*p 34*
71. _D_*p 36*
72. _A_*p 64*
73. _A_*p 63*
74. _C_*p 45*
75. _A_*p 46*
76. _A_*p 56*
77. _B_*p 56*
78. _A_*p 56*
79. _A_*p 55*
80. _B_*p 65*
81. _C_*p 33*
82. _B_*p 41*
83. _C_*p 65*
84. _A_*p 26*
85. _B_*p 36*
86. _D_*p 53*
87. _B_*p 54*
88. _B_*p 41*
89. _D_*p 53*
90. _A_*p 52*
91. _D_*p 53*
92. _A_*p 65*
93. _A_*p 48*

94. _A_*p 64*
95. _A_*p 65*
96. _D_*p 63*
97. _B_*p 65*
98. _B_*p 65–66*
99. _D_*p 65*
100. _A_*p 66*
101. _C_*p 64*
102. _B_*p 48*
103. _B_*p 66*
104. _D_*p 66*
105. _A_*p 67*
106. _D_*p 63*
107. _B_*p 66*
108. _A_*p 67*
109. _A_*p 64*
110. _A_*p 15*
111. _C_*p 16*
112. _A_*p 87*
113. _C_*p 77*
114. _A_*p 77*
115. _C_*p 77*
116. _D_*p 18*
117. _A_*p 15*
118. _D_*p 18*
119. _D_*p 15*
120. _D_*p 71*
121. _C_*p 71*
122. _D_*p 71*
123. _A_*p 71*
124. _A_*p 71*

125. _B_p 72
126. _B_p 72
127. _C_p 71
128. _A_p 72
129. _D_p 71
130. _A_p 36
131. _D_p 71
132. _D_p 71
133. _C_p 73
134. _B_p 72
135. _A_p 76
136. _D_p 81
137. _A_p 89
138. _B_p 80
139. _A_p 75, 79
140. _A_p 80
141. _C_p 81

142. _D_p 78
143. _B_p 75
144. _B_p 79
145. _A_p 79
146. _B_p 80
147. _B_p 80
148. _B_p 80
149. _B_p 80
150. _D_p 75
151. _C_p 78
152. _A_p 18
153. _B_p 78
154. _B_p 17
155. _C_p 76
156. _C_p 86
157. _C_p 87

158. _D_p 85
159. _C_p 86
160. _A_p 87
161. _C_p 88
162. _C_p 88
163. _A_p 88
164. _A_p 88
165. _D_p 89
166. _B_p 90
167. _A_p 90
168. _D_p 90
169. _D_p 87
170. _B_p 75–78
171. _C_p 87
172. _A_p 89
173. _A_p 64

174. _B_p 71
175. _D_p 87
176. _D_p 87
177. _B_p 87
178. _C_p 48–50
179. _B_p 48
180. _B_p 48
181. _D_p 48–50
182. _D_p 48
183. _B_p 48–50
184. _D_p 48–50
185. _A_p 48–50
186. _C_p 48–50
187. _D_p 48–50
188. _C_p 48–50
189. _A_p 48–50

CHAPTER 2

Pulmonary Practice Exam

CHAPTER 3 ————————————————

Neurology Practice Exam

1. _A_p 158	32. _C_p 194	63. _A_p 202	94. _D_p 167
2. _C_p 158–159	33. _C_p 214	64. _C_p 221	95. _A_p 167
3. _B_p 158	34. _A_p 194	65. _A_p 177	96. _D_p 187
4. _D_p 159	35. _B_p 215	66. _A_p 225	97. _D_p 186
5. _A_p 159	36. _D_p 194	67. _C_p 227–228	98. _D_p 185
6. _B_p 161	37. _A_p 196	68. _D_p 209–210	99. _D_p 186
7. _D_p 160	38. _B_p 195	69. _C_p 209	100. _B_p 186
8. _A_p 161	39. _A_p 213	70. _A_p 210	101. _B_p 187
9. _A_p 161	40. _C_p 213	71. _D_p 210	102. _D_p 194
10. _B_p 163	41. _C_p 213	72. _D_p 222	103. _D_p 167
11. _D_p 163	42. _D_p 214	73. _B_p 217	104. _B_p 167
12. _C_p 163	43. _B_p 213	74. _B_p 205	105. _C_
13. _B_p 164	44. _D_p 217	75. _C_p 205	106. _C_p 192
14. _D_p 164	45. _C_p 339	76. _A_p 222	107. _A_p 220
15. _C_p 164	46. _A_p 165	77. _D_p 227–228	108. _C_p 213
16. _A_p 160	47. _D_p 179	78. _B_p 205–206	109. _B_p 220
17. _B_p 160	48. _D_p 179	79. _B_p 206	110. _A_p 214, 220
18. _B_p 165	49. _D_p 220	80. _A_p 203	111. _C_p 214, 220
19. _C_p 177	50. _C_p 161	81. _D_p 186	112. _D_
20. _A_p 180	51. _D_p 213	82. _C_p 186	113. _D_p 222
21. _B_p 179	52. _D_p 213	83. _C_p 203	114. _A_p 217
22. _B_p 165	53. _D_p 163	84. _A_p 201	115. _C_p 224
23. _A_p 162	54. _D_p 192	85. _C_p 202	116. _D_p 213
24. _C_p 183	55. _C_p 170, 192	86. _D_p 206	117. _C_p 162
25. _D_p 184	56. _B_p 192	87. _B_p 206	118. _C_p 162
26. _B_p 186	57. _D_p 217	88. _D_p 213	119. _A_p 202
27. _B_p 186	58. _D_p 217	89. _B_p 176–177	120. _C_p 211
28. _D_p 187	59. _A_p 215	90. _A_p 177	121. _A_p 212
29. _A_p 187	60. _C_p 163	91. _C_p 179	122. _C_p 176–177
30. _A_p 189	61. _D_p 220	92. _A_p 184	123. _A_p 193
31. _B_p 167	62. _D_p 219	93. _A_p 186	124. _B_p 194

CHAPTER 4 —————————————

Gastroenterology Practice Exam

1. _B_ *p 231*
2. _A_ *p 169, 235*
3. _D_ *p 232*
4. _B_ *p 232*
5. _A_ *p 232*
6. _D_ *p 232*
7. _C_ *p 234*
8. _B_ *p 235*
9. _A_ *p 234*
10. _A_ *p 234*
11. _B_ *p 234*
12. _A_ *p 235*
13. _C_ *p 234*
14. _D_ *p 235*
15. _D_ *p 234*
16. _B_ *p 236*
17. _A_ *p 234*
18. _C_
19. _B_ *p 239*
20. _D_ *p 239, 253*

21. _B_ *p 239*
22. _B_ *p 253*
23. _D_ *p 239*
24. _C_ *p 239*
25. _A_ *p 238*
26. _C_ *p 239*
27. _B_ *p 239*
28. _A_ *p 236–239*
29. _A_ *p 236*
30. _B_ *p 236*
31. _C_ *p 241*
32. _B_ *p 241*
33. _D_ *p 242*
34. _D_ *p 242–243*
35. _C_ *p 243–245*
36. _A_ *p 244–245*
37. _C_ *p 236*
38. _A_ *p 245*
39. _D_ *p 246–247*
40. _A_ *p 248*

41. _A_ *p 247*
42. _C_
43. _A_ *p 251*
44. _B_ *p 251*
45. _B_ *p 255*
46. _B_ *p 255*
47. _A_ *p 255*
48. _A_ *p 255*
49. _D_ *p 256*
50. _C_ *p 257*
51. _A_ *p 258*
52. _B_ *p 257*
53. _D_ *p 258*
54. _D_ *p 259*
55. _D_ *p 259*
56. _A_ *p 261, 263*
57. _B_ *p 251*
58. _B_ *p 262*
59. _A_ *p 262*

60. _B_ *p 262*
61. _B_ *p 265*
62. _D_ *p 266*
63. _D_ *p 266*
64. _C_ *p 267*
65. _D_ *p 267*
66. _A_ *p 268*
67. _B_ *p 269*
68. _C_ *p 268–269*
69. _C_ *p 269*
70. _A_ *p 269*
71. _D_ *p 269*
72. _A_ *p 271*
73. _C_ *p 272*
74. _A_ *p 273*
75. _D_ *p 273*
76. _B_ *p 274*
77. _C_ *p 274*
78. _D_ *p 274*

CHAPTER 5 _____

Renal Practice Exam

1. _B_ *p 287*
2. _D_ *p 287*
3. _A_ *p 290*
4. _B_ *p 288*
5. _C_ *p 287*
6. _B_ *p 293*
7. _A_ *p 293*
8. _C_ *p 294*
9. _A_ *p 295*
10. _B_ *p 295*
11. _B_ *p 304*
12. _A_ *p 297–316*
13. _C_ *p 297*
14. _D_ *p 303–304*
15. _C_ *p 305*
16. _A_ *p 316*
17. _D_ *p 307*
18. _A_ *p 303–311*
19. _A_ *p 309*

20. _A_ *p 299*
21. _B_ *p 297*
22. _B_ *p 297*
23. _C_ *p 297*
24. _B_ *p 296*
25. _C_ *p 299*
26. _A_ *p 316*
27. _A_ *p 316*
28. _A_ *p 316*
29. _C_ *p 300*
30. _D_ *p 300–301*
31. _A_ *p 301*
32. _D_ *p 301*
33. _B_ *p 303*
34. _A_ *p 300*
35. _A_ *p 301–302*
36. _A_ *p 297*
37. _C_ *p 303–304*
38. _B_ *p 304*

39. _C_ *p 304*
40. _A_ *p 305*
41. _C_ *p 297*
42. _A_ *p 305*
43. _B_ *p 305*
44. _C_ *p 306*
45. _D_ *p 306*
46. _C_ *p 306*
47. _C_ *p 307–309*
48. _D_ *p 307*
49. _B_ *p 307–309*
50. _B_ *p 309*
51. _C_ *p 309*
52. _C_ *p 309*
53. _A_ *p 309–310*
54. _D_ *p 309*
55. _C_ *p 310*
56. _B_ *p 311*
57. _A_ *p 311*

58. _C_ *p 300, 311*
59. _B_ *p 311*
60. _A_ *p 315–316*
61. _A_ *p 315*
62. _C_ *p 303–304*
63. _B_ *p 311*
64. _B_ *p 311*
65. _A_ *p 78, 315–316*
66. _A_ *p 78*
67. _C_ *p 316*
68. _C_ *p 316*
69. _C_ *p 339–340*
70. _B_ *p 316*
71. _B_ *p 319*
72. _D_ *p 324–325*
73. _B_ *p 324–325*
74. _A_ *p 324–325*
75. _D_ *p 324–325*

CHAPTER 6 ⸻

Endocrine Practice Exam

CHAPTER 7

Immunology and Hematology Practice Exam

1. _C_p 373
2. _C_p 372–373
3. _D_p 373
4. _A_p 368–369
5. _B_p 372
6. _D_p 372
7. _C_p 373
8. _A_p 368–369
9. _C_p 373–374
10. _D_p 372
11. _B_p 405
12. _D_p 405
13. _C_p 400
14. _C_p 373
15. _D_p 373
16. _C_p 400

17. _D_p 400
18. _D_p 373–374
19. _B_p 372–373
20. _D_p 404
21. _A_p 404
22. _A_p 400
23. _B_p 404
24. _A_p 407–408
25. _D_p 372
26. _D_p 409
27. _B_p 409
28. _C_p 408–409
29. _D_p 409
30. _A_p 407
31. _D_p 405–406

32. _C_p 406
33. _B_p 405
34. _B_p 407
35. _C_p 407
36. _A_p 388
37. _D_p 388
38. _A_p 407
39. _A_p 407
40. _B_p 393
41. _D_p 390
42. _A_p 392
43. _C_p 388
44. _B_p 408
45. _D_p 409
46. _C_p 409

47. _B_p 409
48. _D_p 398
49. _A_p 357
50. _A_p 387
51. _C_p 388
52. _B_p 409
53. _C_p 368
54. _C_p 374
55. _B_p 370
56. _D_p 371
57. _D_p 388–389
58. _B_p 390
59. _D_p 404
60. _A_p 372
61. _B_p 378

Multisystem Organ Dysfunction Practice Exam

1. _B_ _p 431_
2. _C_ _p 431_
3. _B_ _p 431_
4. _C_ _p 436_
5. _A_ _p 436–437_
6. _A_ _p 436_
7. _C_ _p 435_
8. _D_ _p 414_
9. _C_ _p 414_
10. _D_ _p 418–419_
11. _D_ _p 416_

12. _C_ _p 420_
13. _B_ _p 436_
14. _A_ _p 420_
15. _B_ _p 420_
16. _C_ _p 420_
17. _C_ _p 420_
18. _B_ _p 414–415_
19. _D_ _p 416_
20. _B_ _p 414–415_
21. _B_ _p 417_
22. _B_ _p 418_

23. _A_ _p 418_
24. _D_ _p 438_
25. _B_ _p 433_
26. _B_ _p 429_
27. _D_ _p 422, 424_
28. _A_ _p 423_
29. _B_ _p 423_
30. _C_ _p 414_
31. _A_ _p 421_
32. _C_ _p 431_
33. _A_ _p 436_

34. _C_ _p 435_
35. _D_ _p 435–436_
36. _C_ _p 437_
37. _D_ _p 436_
38. _C_ _p 436_
39. _B_ _p 436_
40. _B_ _p 437_
41. _C_ _p 437–438_
42. _D_ _p 435–436_
43. _C_ _p 437_
44. _A_ _p 432_

CHAPTER 9

Comprehensive Practice Exam—1

1. _B_*p 15*
2. _B_*p 15*
3. _C_*p 48*
4. _A_*p 66*
5. _C_*p 69–70*
6. _A_*p 71*
7. _A_*p 95–98*
8. _B_*p 315, 316*
9. _C_*p 316*
10. _B_*p 214*
11. _D_*p 38*
12. _D_*p 144*
13. _B_*p 144*
14. _D_*p 405*
15. _D_*p 304*
16. _B_*p 305*
17. _D_*p 16*
18. _C_*p 144*
19. _B_*p 144*
20. _C_*p 368*
21. _C_*p 306*
22. _C_*p 307*
23. _A_*p 16*
24. _D_*p 123*
25. _C_*p 283*
26. _C_*p 48*
27. _B_*p 78*
28. _C_*p 78*
29. _D_*p 435*

30. _C_*p 431*
31. _D_*p 436*
32. _D_*p 48*
33. _A_*p 66*
34. _A_*p 139*
35. _C_*p 138, 139*
36. _C_*p 254*
37. _B_*p 63*
38. _C_*p 63*
39. _D_*p 137*
40. _A_*p 137*
41. _A_*p 435*
42. _D_*p 88*
43. _A_*p 89*
44. _D_*p 130*
45. _C_*p 259*
46. _D_*p 213*
47. _A_*p 217*
48. _B_*p 14*
49. _C_*p 131*
50. _A_*p 313*
51. _B_*p 316*
52. _A_*p 15*
53. _B_*p 21*
54. _A_*p 414*
55. _B_*p 420*
56. _A_*p 142*
57. _B_*p 361*
58. _B_*p 361*

59. _D_*p 72*
60. _D_*p 125*
61. _C_*p 395*
62. _A_*p 373*
63. _A_*p 361*
64. _A_*p 16*
65. _A_*p 115*
66. _D_*p 277*
67. _C_*p 17*
68. _B_*p 329*
69. _B_*p 20*
70. _B_*p 117*
71. _C_*p 306*
72. _B_*p 340*
73. _B_*p 340*
74. _D_*p 49*
75. _D_*p 71*
76. _C_*p 129*
77. _A_*p 248*
78. _A_*p 253*
79. _D_*p 195*
80. _B_*p 196*
81. _B_*p 405*
82. _A_*p 12*
83. _B_*p 129*
84. _C_*p 129*
85. _A_*p 388*
86. _D_*p 383*
87. _D_*p 8*

88. _C_*p 86*
89. _D_*p 269*
90. _B_*p 395*
91. _A_*p 396*
92. _B_*p 11*
93. _A_*p 139*
94. _C_*p 425*
95. _D_*p 186*
96. _C_*p 70*
97. _D_*p 123*
98. _B_*p 224*
99. _D_*p 278*
100. _B_*p 279*
101. _A_*p 53*
102. _C_*p 70*
103. _A_*p 71*
104. _B_*p 401*
105. _D_*p 432*
106. _D_*p 48*
107. _D_*p 132*
108. _C_*p 87*
109. _D_*p 87*
110. _A_*p 406*
111. _C_*p 406*
112. _C_*p 65*
113. _A_*p 130*
114. _D_*p 304*
115. _C_*p 305*
116. _A_*p 53*

117. _C_ _p_ 107
118. _C_ _p_ 14
119. _B_ _p_ 67
120. _D_ _p_ 348
121. _C_ _p_ 348
122. _D_ _p_ 36
123. _A_ _p_ 132
124. _A_ _p_ 267
125. _B_ _p_ 306
126. _A_ _p_ 63
127. _A_ _p_ 71
128. _B_ _p_ 72
129. _D_ _p_ 180
130. _B_ _p_ 194
131. _C_ _p_ 57
132. _D_ _p_ 142
133. _A_ _p_ 300
134. _D_ _p_ 431
135. _D_ _p_ 436
136. _C_ _p_ 55
137. _A_ _p_ 149

138. _D_ _p_ 283
139. _A_ _p_ 375
140. _C_ _p_ 187
141. _D_ _p_ 65
142. _C_ _p_ 151
143. _A_ _p_ 50
144. _B_ _p_ 184
145. _D_ _p_ 400
146. _D_ _p_ 79
147. _A_ _p_ 80
148. _A_ _p_ 143
149. _D_ _p_ 215
150. _C_ _p_ 50
151. _B_ _p_ 64
152. _B_ _p_ 404
153. _A_ _p_ 130
154. _D_ _p_ 71
155. _C_ _p_ 206
156. _C_ _p_ 64
157. _A_ _p_ 438
158. _D_ _p_ 438

159. _B_ _p_ 268
160. _C_ _p_ 69
161. _D_ _p_ 66
162. _B_ _p_ 222
163. _C_ _p_ 137
164. _B_ _p_ 139
165. _C_ _p_ 420
166. _B_ _p_ 80
167. _B_ _p_ 90
168. _A_ _p_ 137
169. _A_ _p_ 269
170. _D_ _p_ 269
171. _C_ _p_ 15
172. _B_ _p_ 436
173. _D_ _p_ 15
174. _C_ _p_ 214
175. _A_ _p_ 217
176. _B_ _p_ 138
177. _A_ _p_ 15
178. _A_ _p_ 69
179. _C_ _p_ 348

180. _D_ _p_ 71
181. _A_ _p_ 54
182. _B_ _p_ 304
183. _D_ _p_ 124
184. _A_ _p_ 124
185. _D_ _p_ 115
186. _C_ _p_ 39
187. _C_ _p_ 194
188. _D_ _p_ 194
189. _A_ _p_ 142
190. _A_ _p_ 142
191. _B_ _p_ 436
192. _D_ _p_ 71
193. _B_ _p_ 192
194. _A_ _p_ 359
195. _D_ _p_ 431
196. _A_ _p_ 203
197. _B_ _p_ 203
198. _C_ _p_ 133, 134
199. _D_ _p_ 325
200. _D_ _p_ 72

CHAPTER 10

Comprehensive Practice Exam—2

1. _C_p 69
2. _B_p 71
3. _A_p 313
4. _D_p 316
5. _D_p 213
6. _A_p 217
7. _A_p 50
8. _A_p 313
9. _D_p 123
10. _A_p 126
11. _C_p 126
12. _B_p 152
13. _D_p 152
14. _D_p 67
15. _A_p 66
16. _B_p 248
17. _C_p 248
18. _C_p 431
19. _A_p 436
20. _A_p 368
21. _D_p 369
22. _D_p 14
23. _C_p 71
24. _D_p 108
25. _D_p 280
26. _C_p 48
27. _C_p 50
28. _C_p 437
29. _B_p 436

30. _A_p 70
31. _B_p 71
32. _C_p 213
33. _C_p 217
34. _D_p 340
35. _A_p 340
36. _B_p 130
37. _D_p 405
38. _A_p 406
39. _D_p 436
40. _B_p 436
41. _B_p 15
42. _A_p 130
43. _D_p 15
44. _C_p 258
45. _D_p 262
46. _A_p 66
47. _D_p 78
48. _A_p 78
49. _D_p 115
50. _D_p 438
51. _C_p 48
52. _B_p 66
53. _A_p 64
54. _D_p 128
55. _A_p 234
56. _C_p 179
57. _A_p 179
58. _B_p 16

59. _C_p 115
60. _D_p 431
61. _B_p 436
62. _A_p 128
63. _D_p 15
64. _A_p 15
65. _B_p 435
66. _D_p 436
67. _C_p 130
68. _C_p 16
69. _B_p 71
70. _D_p 258
71. _C_p 257
72. _A_p 130
73. _B_p 119
74. _A_p 64
75. _B_p 65
76. _B_p 117
77. _B_p 15
78. _C_p 78
79. _D_p 133
80. _D_p 32
81. _C_p 78
82. _A_p 80
83. _C_p 115
84. _D_p 70
85. _C_p 361
86. _B_p 361
87. _A_p 20

88. _C_p 65
89. _C_p 131
90. _A_p 15
91. _D_p 405
92. _D_p 436
93. _A_p 65
94. _A_p 184
95. _D_p 21
96. _D_p 71
97. _A_p 227
98. _B_p 227
99. _D_p 132
100. _B_p 262
101. _A_p 124
102. _C_p 47
103. _A_p 55
104. _C_p 142
105. _B_p 142
106. _D_p 15
107. _B_p 315
108. _C_p 316
109. _D_p 267
110. _D_p 149
111. _B_p 71
112. _B_p 142
113. _D_p 435
114. _C_p 54
115. _A_p 431
116. _C_p 437